Treating Alcohol Dependence
Second Edition

TREATING ALCOHOL DEPENDENCE

A Coping Skills Training Guide

SECOND EDITION

Peter M. Monti
Ronald M. Kadden
Damaris J. Rohsenow
Ned L. Cooney
David B. Abrams

Foreword by G. Alan Marlatt

THE GUILFORD PRESS
New York   London

Printed in the United States of America

This book is printed on acid-free paper.

Last digit is print number: 9 8 7 6 5 4 3 2 1

Library of Congress Cataloging-in-Publication Data

Treating alcohol dependence: a coping skills training guide / Peter M.
Monti . . . [et al.].—2nd ed.
  p. cm.
Previous edition published in series: Treatment manuals for
practitioners.
Includes bibliographical references and index.
  ISBN 1-57230-793-5 (pbk: alk. paper)
  1. Alcoholism—Treatment. 2. Alcoholics—Rehabilitation. 3. Life
skills. 4. Adjustment (Psychology) I. Monti, Peter M.
  RC565 .M634 2002
  616.86′106—dc21
                                                    2002008926

About the Authors

Peter M. Monti, PhD, is Professor of Medical Science and Director of the Center for Alcohol and Addiction Studies and the Clinical Psychology Internship Consortium at Brown University, Providence, Rhode Island. His research is supported by a Senior Research Scientist Award from the Department of Veterans Affairs and he holds research grants from the National Institute on Alcohol Abuse and Alcoholism, the National Institute on Drug Abuse, and the Department of Veterans Affairs. Widely published, Dr. Monti is coauthor of *Nicotine Dependence: An Evidence-Based Clinical Guide* (Guilford Press, forthcoming) and coeditor of *Adolescents, Alcohol, and Substance Abuse: Reaching Teens through Brief Interventions* (Guilford Press, 2001) and *Social Skills Training: A Practical Handbook for Assessment and Treatment* (Guilford Press, 1982). He is a Fellow of the American Psychological Society and the American Psychological Association.

Ronald M. Kadden, PhD, is currently Professor of Psychology in the Department of Psychiatry at the University of Connecticut School of Medicine. His clinical orientation is cognitive-behavioral. He is an attending psychologist in the Alcohol, Drug Abuse, and Psychiatric Day Hospital Program at the UConn Health Center. Dr. Kadden's research focuses on treatment effectiveness for chemical dependence, especially alcohol and marijuana dependence. He has over 60 scientific publications, is a Fellow of the American Psychological Association and the Academy of Behavioral Medicine Research, and is a member of the Research Society on Alcoholism, the Association for Advancement of Behavior Therapy, and the Connecticut Psychological Association.

Damaris J. Rohsenow, PhD, is Professor (Research) of Community Health and Research Director of the Addictive Behaviors Lab at the Center for Alcohol and Addiction Studies at Brown University, and is a Research Career Scientist at the Providence VA Medical Center in Providence, Rhode Island. Her program of research is supported by numerous grants awarded by the National Institute on Alcohol Abuse and Alcoholism, the National Institute on Drug Abuse, the Merit Review program of the Office of Medical Research of the Department of Veterans Affairs, and the Centers for Disease Control and Prevention. Dr. Rohsenow's research ranges from laboratory investigations of mechanisms through controlled clinical trials of newly developed behavioral or pharmacological treatments, as applied to the problems of alcohol dependence, cocaine abuse, and tobacco use.

Ned L. Cooney, PhD, is Associate Professor of Psychiatry at Yale University School of Medicine and Director of Mental Health and Substance Abuse Programs at the Newington Campus of the VA Connecticut Healthcare System. He has conducted research and authored many articles on alcoholism treatment matching, alcohol cue reactivity, and the interaction of alcohol and tobacco dependence. Dr. Cooney is currently Principal Investigator on a project funded by the National Institute on Alcohol Abuse and Alcoholism investigating smoking cessation treatment for alcoholic smokers.

David B. Abrams, PhD, is Professor of Psychiatry and Human Behavior at Brown Medical School/The Miriam Hospital and Director of the Centers for Behavioral and Preventive Medicine. He is interested in understanding the mechanisms underlying addictive behavior to improve treatment, prevention, and inform policy. He is Principal Investigator of many grant awards from agencies of the National Institutes of Health, including a Special Center of Research Excellence from the National Cancer Institute on nicotine dependence across generations and from the National Institute on Alcohol Abuse and Alcoholism on motivating alcoholics for smoking cessation. Dr. Abrams is President of the Society of Behavioral Medicine, Co-director of the Robert Wood Johnson Foundation's Tobacco Etiology Research Network, and a member of the Board of Scientific Advisors of the National Cancer Institute. He is a Fellow of the American Psychological Association and the Society of Behavioral Medicine and holds a Distinguished Scientist Award from the Society of Behavioral Medicine.

Acknowledgments

We wish to thank many individuals for their work that has contributed to this book. The initial drafts of some of the sessions in Chapters 3 and 4 were developed in collaboration with Drs. James Curran, Donald Corriveau, William Norman, Toy Caldwell-Colbert, Steven Hayes, Jody Binkoff, Sue Hagerman, Gail Beck, Roger Pinto, Richard Brown, John Elder, Anthony Rubonis, Suzy Gulliver, Elise Kabela, and Mark Litt. Thanks go to all of these individuals.

We also thank those authors of clinical handbooks and other manuals whose ideas and techniques were sometimes adapted for our work with alcoholics. We have attempted to acknowledge these contributions in the text.

We are grateful to the many students and therapists who made use of these materials in our clinical trials and who provided us with much valuable feedback. We also wish to thank Kathy Bennett and Priscilla Terry for their patience and hard work in preparing the manuscript.

Our work was supported in part by grants from the Veterans Administration Merit Review; National Heart, Lung and Blood Institute; National Cancer Institute; National Institute on Drug Abuse; National Institute on Alcohol Abuse and Alcoholism; the Alcohol Research Center at the University of Connecticut; and by Career Research Scientist awards from the Department of Veterans Affairs.

Our greatest respect goes to the many hundreds of patients fighting alcohol dependence who have managed to cope successfully with their disorder and resume happy and productive lives for themselves and with their families. These individuals provide role models for other patients, and for their children as well.

It is with love and appreciation that we dedicate this book to Sylvia Monti, Marion Wachtenheim, Renana Kadden, Judith Lifshitz Cooney, and Norman Dudziak, Jr.

Foreword

In my foreword to the first edition of this book, published in 1989, I wrote that "this book is the first detailed training manual for skills training with alcohol-dependent individuals. I am impressed with the breadth and depth of the information presented on skills training and how to apply it in various clinical settings." I am pleased to say that my overall evaluation of this new edition is equally positive and enthusiastic. Peter Monti and his colleagues have provided the field with an updated and improved version of their coping skills training guide for treating and preventing relapse of alcohol dependence.

As in the first edition, the primary focus is on training both therapists and clients how to teach and acquire basic coping skills that have been shown to be effective in enhancing treatment maintenance. The book opens with an introductory chapter that provides an updated and comprehensive review of the theoretical underpinnings of the skills training approach. Here, the authors describe the cognitive–social learning model as it applies to both the etiology and treatment of problem drinking and alcoholism. Chapter 1 begins with the acknowledgment of four new important changes in the field since the publication of the first edition: the emergence of managed care and the corresponding reduction in long-term residential treatment programs; the advent of new pharmacological treatments for alcohol dependence; the introduction of motivational enhancement strategies to prepare clients for behavior change; and the upswing in interest in treating clients with comorbid psychiatric disorders. Each of these recent developments is integrated throughout the book in terms of its implications for current treatment programs. The chapter also includes a review of research documenting the effectiveness of the coping skills intervention.

Chapter 2 is a new addition to the original text, and presents valuable information for therapists concerning general treatment considerations. Here, the focus is on both setting the stage for treatment and the nature of the treatment setting. Topics include therapist training, the use of cotherapist teams in group treatment settings, motivational issues (including motivational interviewing with less motivated clients), and incorporating family members into the treatment group. Treatment setting issues include a discussion of conducting skills training programs in partial hospital or day treatment settings, implementation in outpatient settings, and consideration of treatment approaches for both group and individual therapy.

As in the first edition, the core of the new book rests in Chapters 3 and 4 on coping skills training. Chapter 3 is devoted to training in interpersonal and communication skills. A variety of skills are covered in detail, including nonverbal communication, assertiveness, positive feedback, conversation and listening, giving and receiving criticism, drink refusal, resolving relationship problems, and developing social support networks. In Chapter 4, several critical intrapersonal (cognitive and emotional) coping skills are discussed, including managing urges to drink, problem solving, increasing pleasant activities, anger management, dealing with negative thinking, recognizing "seemingly irrelevant decisions" that may lead to relapse, and planning for emergencies.

In both chapters, each coping skill is fully described and presented in a clinically relevant context, including sections on the rationale for using a particular coping skill, specific skills training guidelines, how to model coping and engage in role plays (behavioral rehearsal), and practice exercises. In addition, valuable therapist "Tip Sheets" are included to provide further documentation of techniques.

The final two chapters are both entirely new to this revised edition. Chapter 5 provides an overview of cue exposure treatment combined with urge coping training. Recent research (much of it conducted by Peter Monti and his coworkers at Brown University) documents that exposing clients to alcohol cues as part of the treatment regimen often triggers strong reactivity (both physiological and cognitive), experienced as strong urges or craving to drink. Cue exposure techniques are described, along with a description of urge-specific coping skills. Since urges are frequently precipitated by alcohol cue exposure, therapists are able to teach clients how to cope with urges as they occur "on the spot" in response to alcohol-related stimuli. Individual differences in cue reactivity are also discussed. Chapter 6 is also devoted to a timely topic, and one of growing clinical significance: the treatment of dual diagnosis clients. Both clients and therapists will benefit from this discussion of an integrated approach to working with co-occurring problems of alcohol dependence and various psychiatric disorders. Several common dual diagnosis problems associated with alcohol dependence are described in detail, including co-occurring depression, anxiety, psychosis, and personality disorders. The final section of Chapter 6 is devoted to the treatment of clients with both drinking and smoking dependencies. As many treatment programs for alcoholism also include smoking cessation interventions, this information is especially valuable.

There is increased need for treatment approaches for alcohol dependence that show effectiveness and are "evidence-based," based on evaluations in controlled treatment outcome trials. Although there is no firm evidence that one treatment approach works better than any other for alcohol dependence, the bulk of the outcome studies reviewed in this book provide strong support for a skills training approach. This manual provides a seminal overview of how training clients to engage in effective coping skills can be effective in maintaining treatment gains and preventing relapse. I recommend it highly for both therapists and researchers (including beginning students and experienced professionals) who are actively involved in the treatment of alcohol dependence.

G. ALAN MARLATT, PhD
Addictive Behaviors Research Center, University of Washington

Contents

ONE Introduction, Theoretical Rationale, and Evidence Base 1

Introduction and Overview of This Book, 1
Historical Roots of the Coping Skills Approach to Alcoholism, 2
Social Learning Theory of Alcohol Consumption, 3
Rationale for Coping Skills Training and Cue Exposure Treatment, 8
Evidence Base for Coping Skills Training Approaches, 10
Evidence Base for Cue Exposure Treatment Approaches, 14
Implications of Recent Innovations, 16

TWO General Treatment Considerations: Setting the Stage 19
and Treatment Setting

Introduction, 19
Setting the Stage, 20
Partial Hospital and Day Treatment Considerations, 30
Outpatient and Aftercare Considerations, 31
Individual Treatment Considerations, 39

THREE Coping Skills Training: Part I. Interpersonal Skills 42

General Introduction, 42
Structure of the Sessions, 43
Introducing Clients to This Approach, 44
Session: Nonverbal Communication, 45
Session: Introduction to Assertiveness, 48
Session: Conversation Skills, 50
Session: Giving and Receiving Positive Feedback, 53
Session: Listening Skills, 55
Session: Giving Constructive Criticism, 57
Session: Receiving Criticism about Drinking, 61
Session: Drink Refusal Skills, 65
Session: Resolving Relationship Problems, 66
Session: Developing Social Support Networks, 70

Therapist Tip Sheet: Nonverbal Communication, 73
Reminder Sheet: Nonverbal Communication, 74
Therapist Tip Sheet: Introduction to Assertiveness, 75
Reminder Sheet: Assertiveness, 76
Therapist Tip Sheet: Conversation Skills, 77
Reminder Sheet: Conversation Skills, 78
Therapist Tip Sheet: Giving and Receiving Positive Feedback, 79
Reminder Sheet: Giving and Receiving Positive Feedback, 80
Therapist Tip Sheet: Listening Skills, 81
Reminder Sheet: Listening Skills, 82
Therapist Tip Sheet: Giving Constructive Criticism, 84
Reminder Sheet: Giving Constructive Criticism, 85
Therapist Tip Sheet: Receiving Criticism about Drinking, 86
Reminder Sheet: Receiving Criticism about Drinking, 87
Therapist Tip Sheet: Drink Refusal Skills, 88
Reminder Sheet: Drink Refusal Skills, 89
Therapist Tip Sheet: Resolving Relationship Problems, 90
Reminder Sheet: Resolving Relationship Problems, 91
Therapist Tip Sheet: Developing Social Support Networks, 92
Reminder Sheet: Developing Social Support Networks, 93

FOUR Coping Skills Training: Part II. Intrapersonal Skills 95

General Introduction, 95
Session: Managing Urges to Drink, 96
Session: Problem Solving, 99
Session: Increasing Pleasant Activities, 102
Session: Anger Management, 104
Session: Managing Negative Thinking, 108
Session: Seemingly Irrelevant Decisions, 113
Session: Planning for Emergencies, 115

Therapist Tip Sheet: Managing Urges to Drink, 117
Reminder Sheet: Managing Urges, 118
Therapist Tip Sheet: Problem Solving, 119
Reminder Sheet: Problem Solving, 120
Therapist Tip Sheet: Increasing Pleasant Activities, 121
Reminder Sheet: Increasing Pleasant Activities, 122
Therapist Tip Sheet: Anger Management, 123
Reminder Sheet: Anger Management, 124
Therapist Tip Sheet: Managing Negative Thinking, 126
Reminder Sheet: Managing Negative Thinking, 127
Therapist Tip Sheet: Seemingly Irrelevant Decisions, 128
Reminder Sheet: Seemingly Irrelevant Decisions, 129
Therapist Tip Sheet: Planning for Emergencies, 130
Reminder Sheet: Planning for Emergencies, 131

FIVE Cue Exposure Treatment with Urge Coping Training 132

Conceptual Overview, 132
Methodological Issues in Conducting Cue Exposure, 133
Assessments, 138

Conducting CET with Urge-Specific Coping Skills Training, 140
Individual Differences in Cue Reactivity, 148
Therapist Tip Sheet: Cue Exposure Treatment Rationale, 155
Therapist Tip Sheet: CET Individual Session 1, 156
Therapist Tip Sheet: CET Individual Sessions after First Session, 159
Reminder Sheet: _____'s Toolbox for Reducing Urges, 162

| SIX | Dual Diagnosis Issues | 163 |

General Introduction, 163
Depression, 166
Anxiety Disorders, 168
Psychotic Disorders, 169
Personality Disorders, 171
Tobacco Dependence Issues, 173

| References | 180 |
| Index | 192 |

ONE

Introduction, Theoretical Rationale, and Evidence Base

Introduction and Overview of This Book   1
Historical Roots of the Coping Skills Approach to Alcoholism   2
Social Learning Theory of Alcohol Consumption   3
Rationale for Coping Skills Training and Cue Exposure Treatment   8
Evidence Base for Coping Skills Training Approaches   10
Evidence Base for Cue Exposure Treatment Approaches   14
Implications of Recent Innovations   16

INTRODUCTION AND OVERVIEW OF THIS BOOK

The field of alcohol treatment has undergone substantial changes since the first edition of this book (Monti, Abrams, Kadden, & Cooney, 1989). Paramount among these are four changes. First, the emergence of managed care has drastically reduced the overall length and intensity of treatment. Although long-term residential care and 28-day intensive treatment programs were commonplace 12 years ago, they have all but disappeared from the treatment landscape except to serve those few individuals who can afford to self-pay. The second change is the emergence of new psychopharmacological interventions and other empirically based and/or technologically driven interventions. A third change involves increased sensitivity to clients' intrinsic motivational level for change and adjusting treatment styles to optimize motivation for change (Miller & Rollnick, 2002). A fourth change is the increasing concern about clients with comorbid psychiatric disorders.

Accordingly, this new edition presents a streamlined version of our original treatment program. We give the new psychopharmacological interventions special emphasis at the end of this chapter. Readers will particularly note increased flexibility in the protocols in

1

Chapters 3 and 4. Empirically based cue exposure treatment (CET) is described in Chapter 5. The issue of motivation for change is discussed in this chapter and in Chapter 2. Adaptation of coping skills treatment for clients with comorbid psychopathology is addressed in Chapter 6.

As with the first edition of *Treating Alcohol Dependence*, we have been guided in our work by a cognitive–social learning perspective on alcohol use and abuse. The comprehensive coping skills treatment program presented herein follows directly from this model. Its central tenet is that through a variety of learning techniques (behavioral rehearsal, modeling, cognitive restructuring, didactic instruction, cue exposure with or without coping skills training), individuals and their social networks can be taught to use alternative methods of coping with the demands of living without relying on addictive substances.

The skills that constitute the core of this book were designed for clients diagnosed as alcohol dependent according to the fourth edition of the *Diagnostic and Statistical Manual of Mental Disorders* (DSM-IV; American Psychiatric Association, 1994). However, clients diagnosed as alcohol abusers, or individuals with less severe drinking problems, can also benefit from many of the components presented in this book. Indeed, adolescents who drink excessively have also benefited from modifications of our treatment protocols adapted to their special needs (e.g., Kaminer, Burleson, & Goldberger, 2001; Waldron, Brody, & Slesnick, 2001). Furthermore, given the assumption that addictive behavior is related to difficulties in coping, the skills training program offered herein has also been adopted and proven effective with other substances of abuse (e.g., cocaine; Monti, Rohsenow, Michalec, Martin, & Abrams, 1997).

In this first chapter, we briefly review the historical roots of the coping skills approach to alcoholism and lay out the rationale for both the coping skills and cue exposure treatment approaches. Next, we review the evidence base for both approaches, administered individually as well as combined. Finally, we discuss implications of some of the more recent innovations, including pharmacotherapy.

Chapter 2 reviews general treatment considerations that have evolved and matured, along with the authors themselves, as the field has advanced. Chapters 3 and 4 present the core inter- and intrapersonal skills training components as we have tailored and refined them over the past 12 years. This core is interwoven with clinical examples and anecdotes. We trust that our clinical program has benefited from the many clinical trials conducted over the past decade. Chapters 5 and 6 are entirely new additions to the book and deal with cue exposure treatment and dual diagnosis issues, respectively.

HISTORICAL ROOTS OF THE COPING SKILLS APPROACH TO ALCOHOLISM

The techniques, principles, and approaches to alcohol dependence outlined in this book are derived in part from a model that construes addictive behavior as a habitual, maladaptive way of coping with stress. Major life events; everyday hassles; family, work, and community concerns; and individual lifestyle are all instances of the regularly encountered "stressors" that must be resolved. The resultant strain placed on an individual is also influenced by biological/genetic vulnerability to stressors, behavioral deficits or excesses that are a result of an individual's social learning history, and acute situational demands. Thus, the interaction of various biopsychosocial factors is crucial to understanding the reasons for abuse.

"Stress" may be defined as an "adaptational relationship" (Marlatt, 1985b) between an individual and a situational demand (stressor). Accordingly, the conceptual framework that we adopt views stress as resulting from an imbalance between environmental demands and an individual's resources (Shiffman & Wills, 1985; Wills & Shiffman, 1985). "Coping" is an attempt to meet the demand in a way that restores balance or equilibrium. If the individual does not have adequate coping skills in his/her repertoire to meet the demand, then alcohol use may be an attempt to restore a perception of equilibrium (to cope).

Social learning theory (SLT) acknowledges the role of biological and genetic factors in alcohol dependence. Although it is true that alcoholism runs in families, SLT holds that this phenomenon can best be understood by considering the interaction between genetic influences and psychosocial factors (Abrams & Wilson, 1986). The most salient finding to emerge over the past generation of genetic alcohol research is that genetic factors contribute to individual differences in alcohol-relevant behaviors (McGue, 1999). Both twin and adoption studies have supported the notion of genetic influences on alcoholism risk, with especially compelling findings for men. It should be noted however, that evidence also reveals that sociocultural influences are critically important in genetically predisposed individuals. This suggests that changes in social attitudes and behavior by and toward individuals at high risk for alcoholism can alter both the occurrence and course of the disorder. Genetic vulnerability appears to interact with psychosocial factors, resulting in either good coping with less likelihood of alcohol abuse, or in coping skills deficits that require explicit skills training for remediation.

The SLT model of alcohol abuse is derived from the principles of experimental, social, and cognitive psychology. It has also been referred to as the "addictive behavior model" of alcohol use (Marlatt & Gordon, 1985). The major assumption is that if clients take responsibility for learning new behaviors, they can learn to better manage their genetic and social learning vulnerabilities.

SOCIAL LEARNING THEORY OF ALCOHOL CONSUMPTION

In an early formulation of SLT, Bandura (1969) stated that "alcoholics are people who have acquired, through differential reinforcement and modeling experiences, alcohol consumption as a widely generalized dominant response to aversive stimulation" (p. 536). According to Bandura (1977, 1997), SLT emphasizes cognitive mediational factors in the explanation of learning and behavior. The theory postulates that an individual's expectations about alcohol's effects will influence the likelihood of drinking, as well as behavior when intoxicated. SLT suggests that drinking is acquired and maintained by reinforcement, modeling, conditioned responding, expectations about alcohol's effects, and physical dependence.

Since its beginnings, SLT has generated much basic and clinical research on alcohol use and abuse. Comprehensive reviews (Abrams & Niaura, 1987; Maisto, Carey, & Bradizza, 1999) of this research have identified a set of principles that form a comprehensive version of an SLT of alcohol use and dependence. Because the core of this book reflects the application of several of these principles, we review those that are most pertinent and provide selected examples.

One principle of SLT embodies the developmental notion that learning to drink occurs as part of growing up in a particular culture in which the social influences of family and peers shape the behaviors, beliefs, and expectancies of young people concerning alcohol. Youthful drinking is influenced by the modeling of alcohol consumption; the creation of specific expectations of the benefits of drinking via media portrayals of sexual prowess, power, and success; and social reinforcement from peer groups. In support of this principle, the attitudes and behaviors of parents regarding alcohol appear to be strong predictors of adolescent drinking (Barnes, 1977; O'Leary, O'Leary, & Donovan, 1976). However, the relationship to parental behavior is complex. Conflicting parental attitudes toward alcohol are related to excessive youthful drinking (Jackson & Connor, 1953), and the children of abstainers with fixed and extreme attitudes toward temperance are at increased risk for developing problems (Wittman, 1939).

Marlatt and his associates have studied the effects of peer modeling on drinking for more than two decades. In an early report, Caudill and Marlatt (1975), studying heavy-drinking college students, showed that those who were exposed to a heavy-drinking model drank more than those exposed to either a light-drinking model or no model at all. Other studies have shown that modeling effects are influenced by gender and drinking history (Lied & Marlatt, 1979), by the nature of the interaction between drinking partners (Collins, Parks, & Marlatt, 1985), and by the setting in which drinking occurs (Strickler, Dobbs, & Maxwell, 1979). The overall results of the modeling phenomenon are robust. This knowledge has served as the basis for a college student drinking intervention pioneered by Marlatt and his colleagues, in which normative information is given about drinking on campuses (Miller, Kilmer, Kim, Weingardt, & Marlatt, 2001). This approach is reported to be highly successful (Marlatt et al., 1999).

Modeling techniques are used therapeutically in the skills training program described in this book for teaching general and alcohol-specific coping skills. As each new skill is introduced, the therapists demonstrate the performance of the skill. Other potential sources of modeling influences are group members, as well as relatives (when relatives are included in treatment).

An important effect of both parental and peer modeling may be the development of internalized expectancies for alcohol effects. Indeed, Biddle, Bank, and Marlin (1980) suggest that modeled behaviors get translated into expectancies, which are more important direct determinants of drinking than the modeling itself. The phenomena of alcohol-related expectancies and their effect on drinking have been studied extensively (e.g., Marlatt & Rohsenow, 1980), although for the most part with adults. Developmental factors may complicate their effect on teens and lead to different treatment implications (Monti, Colby, & O'Leary, 2001).

Although it is likely that alcohol-related expectancies are first inculcated by parents and peers, other cultural agents, such as the media, are likely to have an influence as well. For example, a child who sees his/her parents reach for a martini or two to ease the stress of a hard day at work, or to enhance their ability to socialize at a party, is likely to have these notions reinforced and generalized when watching alcohol-related scenes on television. Peers may serve as additional models for using alcohol to reduce tension and further reinforce its use to enhance social pleasure. The adolescent who never learns ways to modulate anxiety without alcohol may come to rely increasingly on alcohol to decrease stress in more and more situations, thus increasing the risk for developing alcoholism.

Reinforcement is another central principle of SLT. Alcohol use is strongly influenced by positive reinforcement (e.g., feelings of euphoria or getting "high"; Wills & Shiffman, 1985) or by the expectation of positive reinforcement (Marlatt, 1985b). Alcohol enhances cutaneous and gastric blood flow, and thereby results in a feeling of warmth (Grunberg & Baum, 1985). It may be that some people learn fewer alternative ways to experience positive feelings and sensations; thus, alcohol use develops to serve this need. Social reinforcement is another important potential source of reinforcement for drinking behavior. Negative reinforcement (terminating unpleasant experiences) or the expectation of negative reinforcement may also be a potent factor in developing or maintaining drinking problems, through reduction of tension or negative moods, relief from pain, or release from social inhibitions. Clearly, both the positive and the negative reinforcing results of alcohol consumption should be considered when assessing clients and planning their treatment.

Another important principle involves the role of environmental stimuli or cues, which either may elicit drinking by means of a Pavlovian conditioning mechanism or set the occasion for drinking (operant conditioning). Alcoholics encounter a variety of alcohol-related cues, such as people, places, objects, time periods, and internal states, that have been associated with past drinking. Cues can include the sight and smell of one's favorite alcoholic beverage; places such as bars, beaches, and homes where drinking occurred; mood states such as stress, anger, or wanting to celebrate; certain times, such as the end of work or Friday evening; and people who had been drinking companions. Because alcoholics are asked to avoid drinking cues while in treatment, our clients may first encounter these cues outside of the treatment setting unexpectedly, and with no one present to help them deal with their internal reactions, posing a risk for relapse. Cue exposure treatment (CET) was developed to help clients reduce the strength of the internal reactions and to provide an opportunity to practice use of coping skills while in the state of arousal that these cues generate. CET is derived jointly from two types of theoretical models: classical learning theory models and SLT models of the relationship between alcohol-related cues and relapse.

Classical learning theory models propose that environmental (exteroceptive) or internal (interoceptive) cues associated with drinking in the past can come to elicit conditioned reactions (such as when a dog salivates to the sound of the can opener working), and these reactions may in turn play a role in triggering a relapse to drinking (Monti, Rohsenow, & Hutchison, 2000; Niaura et al., 1988; Rohsenow, Monti, & Abrams, 1995). Debate exists over the exact nature of these responses. One hypothesis is that the responses resemble the conditioned withdrawal that occurs when the alcohol that the body "expects" is not given. Another hypothesis is that the responses are conditioned compensatory responses, that is, physiological responses designed to counteract alcohol's effects (such as increased stimulation to counteract the anticipated sedation from alcohol). A third hypothesis is that conditioned appetitive responses occur, that is, responses similar to those produced by alcohol itself (such as decreased blood pressure), or responses associated with seeking and approaching alcohol (such as arousal to prepare for the activities involved in getting alcohol, and salivation to prepare for ingestion). Current evidence suggests that the conditioned responses to alcohol cues most strongly resemble conditioned appetitive responses (Niaura et al., 1988). Operant learning models add to this formulation by proposing that in the presence of cues, the alcoholic customarily emits a response (usually drinking) designed to decrease aversive reactions and increase pleasurable effects, thus reinforcing the emitted response. These various models suggest that periods of unreinforced exposure to alcohol cues (cue exposure with response prevention) should result in habituation or extinction of the conditioned reactions.

SLT adds to the classical learning model of the role of cues in relapse in several ways (Abrams & Niaura, 1987). First, SLT suggests that the presence of cues can increase the risk of relapse by making the expected effects of alcohol more salient, thereby increasing the alcoholic's desire to drink. Second, alcohol cues can produce both cognitive and psychophysiological reactions that can interfere with the alcoholic's ability to use coping skills. For example, both arousal and increased thoughts about drinking serve to focus attention on the cues, deflecting attention from thoughts about how to cope with urges. Third, alcoholics may have expectancies about their reactions to cue exposure (outcome expectancies) and their ability to cope in the presence of cues (self-efficacy expectancies). Typically, alcoholics expect exposure to cues to be unbearable, and believe their urge to drink will not decrease while cues are present without drinking. The reactions produced by the alcohol cues can undermine the alcoholic's belief that he/she can effectively cope with the situation. On the other hand, the chance to practice use of coping skills while experiencing the interoceptive reactions that result from the presence of alcohol cues (state-dependent learning) can increase the likelihood that the client will be able to use these skills effectively when later encountering cues (Monti et al., 2000). Information processing theory adds that much alcohol seeking can occur automatically outside of conscious awareness, and that urges actually may indicate an attempt to prevent oneself from drinking (Tiffany, 1990). This indicates that increasing awareness of high-risk situations and teaching alternative behaviors will help to disrupt the automatic chain of events that otherwise leads to drinking.

CET may have a beneficial effect as a result of two different mechanisms: through habituation or extinction of responses, and/or through practicing coping skills in the presence of drinking-related cues. For the first of these, treatment might be designed to reduce the intensity of alcoholics' reactions to drinking cues. Learning theory suggests that repeated exposure to a cue while preventing the drinking response should result in habituation (i.e., a decrease in strength of reactions across exposures) or even extinction (i.e., permanent loss) of the conditioned response. As a result, the disruptive effects of alcohol cues on attentional processes and on the ability to use coping skills should be lessened. However, habituation tends to be limited to the specific cues used, so that the reaction might be easily reinstated with a different cue. Therefore, a wide variety of cues are needed in treatment. With respect to the second mechanism, SLT suggests that practice in applying coping skills in the presence of alcohol cues should increase both the effectiveness of these skills when the cues occur and alcoholics' expectancies about their ability to respond effectively. This should make it easier for an alcoholic to cope successfully in the presence of cues after treatment, even when experiencing a strong reaction to them. Internal reactions to alcohol cues should then interfere less with the alcoholic's ability to apply skills in the real world after treatment.

As of this writing, it is still unclear whether the focus of treatment should be more on pure cue exposure or on practicing coping skills in the presence of cues. Until a definitive answer is available, it may be most productive to include both aspects in the treatment package, to maximize the power of the various mechanisms involved in this approach to treatment.

In addition to learning history and contextual cues, SLT emphasizes the importance of current experience, cognitions, and emotions. These immediate determinants of drinking, or "proximal determinants," include antecedents such as environmental cues, the current cognitive–emotional–physiological state of the individual, and the individual's repertoire of coping and problem-solving skills (e.g., drink refusal skills) and expectations (Abrams & Niaura, 1987).

Cognitive factors other than expectancies also play a central role in Bandura's theory, and they are thought to modulate all person–environment interactions. Whether or not a person drinks in a particular situation is determined by both self-efficacy for alternative behaviors and outcome expectations for drinking. "Self-efficacy," an individual's sense that he/she can cope successfully in a particular situation without drinking, is another central SLT principle. A person's confidence that he/she can cope in a specific situation, and his/her estimation of the chances of succeeding, will determine the selection and implementation of coping behaviors. Clinically, clients must develop *strong* and *realistic* confidence that they can cope with life's demands without having to drink. Realistic confidence develops gradually over time, and it is necessary to actually engage in coping behavior in the natural environment to enhance one's sense of mastery. Often, alcoholics in the early phases of treatment have very high confidence that they will "never drink again." This is usually treated with some skepticism by experienced alcohol counselors; these alcoholics are usually unrealistic or overly confident individuals, who have not yet experienced how difficult it is to stay sober, and they may not yet have developed alternative behaviors to use in difficult situations. Gradual exposure to more and more difficult situations, and successful use of coping and avoidance of drinking in these situations, helps one to develop a realistic sense of confidence in his/her ability to cope successfully without drinking. Graduated practice is therefore emphasized, both within treatment sessions and in one's actual environment between treatment sessions.

By way of summarizing the foregoing principles, consider the following example: Imagine a person in a high state of distress because of a recent marital dispute and work pressure. The individual attends a party, where the expectations are to relax and have fun. Several of his/her friends are already drinking and having a good time (modeling influences). Coping will be determined by the individual's general and alcohol-specific coping skills, cue reactivity, and self-efficacy expectations. Self-efficacy percepts will be influenced by the individual's current stress level and history of coping in similar situations. His/her expectations about the short- and long-term effects of drinking on behavior will also be important; that is, the individual may focus on the immediate positive effects of alcohol (e.g., relaxation and euphoria), while ignoring the longer-term negative consequences (e.g., hangover, depression, possible accident). The person may have low self-efficacy about relaxing or socializing without a drink. If drinking is initiated, various reinforcing effects of alcohol may come into play. In summary, a combination of social learning, developmental, situational, cognitive, and biological psychophysiological factors interact. This interaction results in self-efficacy expectations, leading to behavior that can range from abstinence and finding alternatives to drinking on the one hand, to drinking to excess on the other. We feel it is important that both clients and therapists understand and attend to these multiple factors in assessing clients' vulnerabilities that will require treatment.

RATIONALE FOR COPING SKILLS TRAINING AND CUE EXPOSURE TREATMENT

Both coping skills training and CET have theoretical underpinnings in learning theory. As described in the previous section, the SLT approach to alcohol dependence follows a coping deficit model (Bandura, 1969, 1997). In this model, individuals with deficits in skills for coping with any of a number of life situations are at increased risk for excessive alcohol use as a coping response. Social learning-based treatment seeks to improve coping skills as a means of preventing relapse to drinking. CET, another learning theory-based approach, may have a beneficial effect resulting from two distinct mechanisms. The first is based on the assumption that repeated unreinforced exposure will reduce alcohol cue reactivity, which will in turn reduce the likelihood of relapse. The second mechanism is related to the notion that practicing skills in the presence of alcohol cues should increase their effectiveness in the presence of alcohol cues in real life and increase alcoholics' expectancies that they can respond effectively to them without drinking. This section briefly reviews empirical studies that test various theoretical assumptions related to these conceptualizations.

Are Measured Coping Skills Associated with Drinking Outcome?

Alcoholics have been found to differ from nonalcoholics in skills for coping with alcohol-related high-risk situations (Abrams et al., 1991). Litman et al. (1984) used a Coping Behavior Inventory (CBI) to obtain reports of clients' coping strategies; although the CBI did not predict relapse, alcoholics' ratings of the effectiveness of the Positive Thinking and Avoidance factors discriminated continued abstainers from relapsers. Maisto, Connors, and Zywiak (2000) found that changes in the CBI total score from baseline to 6 months predicted drinking outcome at 12 months. Miller, Westerberg, Harris, and Tonigan (1996), in a prospective study of relapse, found that the CBI factor of Positive Thinking was negatively related to relapse. In a cross-sectional study, Moser and Annis (1996) found that continued abstinence after a relapse crisis is related to the number of coping strategies utilized and to the use of active rather than avoidant coping strategies. In another cross-sectional study, relapsers were more likely to report avoidance and wishful thinking, and less likely to use positive self-statements for coping (Wunschel, Rohsenow, Norcross, & Monti, 1993). In the same study, quantity of drinking was lower for clients who reported more use of substitute activities to cope with urges to drink. Chung, Langenbucher, Labouvie, Pandina, and Moos (2001) found that increased behavioral approach coping predicted lower severity of alcohol problems after 12 months, and that a decline in cognitive-avoidance coping predicted both fewer alcohol dependence symptoms and psychosocial difficulties at 12 months. They also found that cognitive-approach coping was a significant factor throughout the follow-up period, but behavioral-approach coping showed significant effects only between 6 and 12 months after treatment.

Jones and Lanyon (1981) found that both general and alcohol-specific skills are correlated with drinking outcome. Similarly, Moggi, Ouimette, Moos, and Finney (1999) found that among dual diagnosis clients, both general and substance-specific coping skills are associated with abstinence. In contrast, Wells, Catalano, Plotnick, Hawkins, and Brattesani (1989) found that certain observer-rated skills for handling drug-related situations, drug-avoidance skills, and thinking about negative consequences when having urges, are associated with less alcohol use among substance abusers following treatment, whereas general social and stress coping skills (e.g., assertiveness, problem solving) were not associated with posttreatment substance use. Another study used observer ratings of skills in both a general social skills role-play test and the Alcohol-Specific Role Play Test (Monti et al., 1990). Skills in the alcohol-specific tasks predicted less frequent drinking at the 6-month follow-up, whereas general skill was unrelated to outcome. Thus, there is some support for the need to learn coping skills within the context of alcohol-specific situations.

The urge-specific coping skills described in Chapter 5 have also been found to be associated with reduced drinking in three studies. In the first small study (Monti et al., 1993), drinking during the 6-month follow-up was lower for those who reported more use of thinking about negative consequences of drinking or positive consequences of sobriety. In the second, larger study (Rohsenow et al., 2001), less drinking during the 12-month follow-up correlated with use of delay, negative consequences, positive consequences, substitute behavior, substitute consumption, and escape/avoidance of high-risk situations but not with relaxation, imagery, mastery messages, or distraction. Complete abstinence was associated with thinking about positive or negative consequences and escape/avoidance. In the third large study (Monti et al., 2001), the mean frequency of use of the five strategies taught in Chapter 5 predicted lower relapse rate and less drinking during the 12 months of follow-up. Thus, these five urge-specific strategies show good support as targets for intervention.

Longabaugh and Morgenstern (1999) examined controlled clinical trials of cognitive-behavioral treatment (CBT) for alcohol dependence to determine whether coping behaviors were more likely following CBT, and whether they covaried with drinking outcomes. Nine studies met scientific criteria for inclusion in their review. Longabaugh and Morgenstern found that some studies provided evidence that coping behaviors increased more with the CBT, and other studies provided evidence that drinking outcomes covaried with level of coping. However, only one of the nine studies provided evidence that a measure of coping differentially changed in the CBT condition *and* covaried with drinking outcome. Methodological weaknesses in many of the studies prevented testing of the complete mediational model. Longabaugh and Morgenstern concluded that research has yet to establish precisely why CBT is an effective treatment for alcohol dependence. Serious attention should be paid in future studies of coping skills training to test the presumed mechanisms of action of CBT adequately.

Although more research is needed on the causal chain relating skills training treatment and drinking outcome, studies of coping skills in alcoholic clients thus far suggest that both general and alcohol-specific coping skills are associated with alcohol abstinence, more abstinence is associated with utilization of a greater number of coping skills, there is an advantage in the use of active rather than avoidant strategies, and there are benefits associated with the use of both cognitive and behavioral strategies. These findings have influenced the development of the content of this coping skills training guide.

Are Elicited Reactions to Cues Associated with Drinking Outcome?

Various studies provide support for the idea that alcohol cues can increase the risk of re-lapse. First, alcoholics who reacted more strongly to the sight and smell of their preferred alcoholic beverage in a controlled assessment also were found to perform a drink refusal role-play more poorly if an alcohol beverage was actually present than if an empty glass was used (Monti, Rohsenow, Colby, & Abrams, 1995). This indicates that alcohol cues can dis-rupt ability to use coping skills even among alcoholics who perform skillfully when the cues are not present. Second, another study showed that alcohol cues interfere with alcoholics' abilities to pay attention to other stimuli (Sayette et al., 1994). This disruption of attention may reduce one's ability to attend to the use of coping skills. Third, alcoholics who reacted more strongly (in terms of increased salivation and being less attentive) when exposed to alcohol cues in a lab early in treatment were found to drink more during the follow-up af-ter treatment (Rohsenow et al., 1994). Increased skin conductance to alcohol cues also predicted more rapid relapse (Drummond & Glautier, 1994). These studies support an information-processing model (Tiffany, 1990) which posits that people with automatic physiological reactions drink more, whereas people with conscious awareness of cues or of their reactions to the cues drink less. Fourth, in another study, urge to drink in the pres-ence of alcohol cues alone did not predict drinking after treatment, but when alcohol cues were presented together with a negative mood induction, alcoholics who reported more de-sire to drink relapsed to alcohol use more quickly (Cooney, Litt, Morse, Bauer, & Gaupp, 1997). This suggests that combining alcohol cues with emotional triggers may be especially important to help alcoholics deal with preventing relapse. However, in another study, urges in response to alcohol cues alone or to alcohol cues after a negative mood induction were equally predictive of drinking more frequently and more heavily during the year after treat-ment (Monti et al., 2001). Clearly, helping alcoholics to reduce or to cope more effectively with their reactions seems warranted.

EVIDENCE BASE FOR COPING SKILLS
TRAINING APPROACHES

In the following section we review the treatment efficacy studies conducted with coping skills training approaches.

Treatment Main Effects

A number of studies have examined the efficacy of cognitive-behavioral coping skills train-ing for alcoholic clients. In an early study, Hedberg and Campbell (1974) found that behav-ioral family counseling that included rehearsal of communication and assertiveness skills was more effective than desensitization, covert sensitization, and aversion therapy in reduc-ing alcohol intake over the next 6 months. Chaney, O'Leary, and Marlatt (1978) provided relapse prevention training in skills for coping with interpersonal situations (such as drink refusal and managing conflicts with other people) and intrapersonal problems (such as coping with negative moods). Clients who received this training experienced subsequent reductions in days of drinking, amount drunk, and length of drinking episodes compared to a discussion control group and a group with no additional treatment, thus supporting the efficacy of the skills training approach. The skills training predicted more rapid responding to role-played high-risk situations, which in turn predicted less drinking.

In a test of one specific aspect of coping skills training, Freedberg and Johnston (1978) found that adding assertiveness training to an inpatient program significantly improved treatment outcome over the inpatient program alone. Oei and Jackson (1980) found that social skills training was superior to supportive therapy for alcoholics, whether provided as individual or group therapy. In a subsequent study, Oei and Jackson (1982) found that social skills training and cognitive restructuring were both effective for alcoholics, and superior to supportive therapy. Furthermore, clients who received cognitive restructuring showed better maintenance of treatment gains at follow-ups. Eriksen, Björnstad, and Götestam (1986) found better drinking outcomes 1 year after social skills training compared to a discussion-group control procedure. Clients who received the skills training drank less and had more sober days, more continuous abstinence, and more working days. In addition, the duration of effects in this study was particularly encouraging. Ferrell and Galassi (1981) also found, at a 2-year follow-up, that clients who had received social skills (assertiveness) training as a treatment adjunct maintained sobriety significantly longer than those who had received human relations training.

In a study comparing two elements of skills training, Monti et al. (1990) found that inpatient alcoholics who received communication skills training (interpersonal skills), with or without family involvement, consumed significantly less alcohol than those who received cognitive-behavioral mood management training (intrapersonal skills) as treatment adjuncts. The communication skills training group showed the most improvement in observer-rated skill, and these skills ratings predicted better outcomes.

Several studies have failed to demonstrate superior outcomes from cognitive-behavioral skills training. Jones, Kanfer, and Lanyon (1982) compared the Chaney et al. (1978) skills training package to standard treatment with alcoholics of higher socioeconomic status, but found that the effects were not superior to those of a group that simply discussed means of handling high-risk situations. This raises an interesting question, which still has not been settled, regarding how much actual practice of skills is required, as opposed simply to identifying high-risk situations and being aware of how to cope with them. One problem that complicates comparisons between the two studies is that the Chaney et al. sample was more impaired than the relatively high-functioning alcoholics in the Jones et al. study. Another problem with comparing the studies is that the control group in the Chaney et al. (1978) study involved only discussing how clients felt in high-risk situations, whereas the comparison group in the Jones et al. (1982) study that did not differ from the coping skills condition discussed concrete solutions to problem situations, as well as barriers to handling them better, thus including some topics also covered as part of coping skills training.

Sanchez-Craig and Walker (1982) provided residents of an alcoholism halfway house with coping skills training focused on goal setting, problem solving, and cognitive coping with urges to drink. They found no differences compared to control procedures (covert sensitization or discussions of goals and problem solving) on any outcome variables up to an 18-month follow-up. Sjoberg and Samsonowitz (1985) found no differences between outpatient skills training and traditional counseling, and Ito, Donovan, and Hall (1988) found that skills training, provided as aftercare, was not different from interpersonal process groups. In a study of the outcomes of clients enrolled in either 12-step-oriented or cognitive-behavioral-oriented inpatient treatment programs, Finney, Noyes, Coutts, and Moos (1998) found that outcomes anticipated to be specific to CBT were actually present among clients who had participated in either the cognitive-behavioral- or 12-step-oriented programs.

Project MATCH was a large, multisite alcoholism treatment trial that compared the effects of 12 sessions of primarily intrapersonal CBT to 12 sessions of 12-step facilitation (TSF) or four sessions of motivational enhancement therapy (MET). Treatment was delivered individually either as low-intensity outpatient treatment or as aftercare treatment following completion of intensive inpatient or outpatient treatment. In general, there were no outcome differences among the three treatments in the Aftercare arm. In the Outpatient arm, however, some modest differences emerged. During the 12-week treatment phase, CBT and TSF clients drank less often than MET clients. MET clients were drinking an average of 20 days throughout the 90-day treatment phase compared with 15 days for CBT and TSF clients. On a Composite Outcome measure, more than 40% of CBT and TSF clients were classified as either abstinent or drinking moderately without problems, compared with 28% of MET clients (Project MATCH Research Group, 1998). Treatment differences faded among outpatients in the year after treatment (Project MATCH research Group, 1997). No enduring clinically significant differences were found among treatments on measures of frequency of drinking, intensity of drinking, or negative consequences. Thus, Project MATCH found that a cognitive-behavioral coping skills individual treatment approach was roughly equivalent to other credible, manual-guided active treatment approaches when provided as the sole outpatient treatment or after successfully completing an intensive program.

Treatment Matching Studies

Some support for the coping skills approach with particular types of clients has also been provided by treatment matching studies. Some matching studies found that group coping skills training (mixed interpersonal and intrapersonal) was more effective than interactional therapy for alcoholics who had high scores on measures of sociopathy and/or psychiatric severity (Kadden, Cooney, Getter, & Litt, 1989; Cooney, Kadden, Litt, & Getter, 1991; Longabaugh et al. 1994). However, Kadden, Litt, Cooney, Kabela, and Getter (2001), in a close replication of the earlier Kadden et al. and Cooney et al. procedures, were unable to reproduce their original matching findings. Another matching study (Rohsenow et al., 1991) found that intrapersonal skills training was effective only for patients with higher education, or lower anxiety or urges to drink, whereas interpersonal skills training was effective regardless of individual differences.

Project MATCH tested the treatment matching hypothesis using CBT, TSF, or MET. Four matching interactions were statistically significant out of 21 that were tested. These significant interactions involved client anger, social support for drinking, severity of alcohol dependence, and global psychopathology. The matching effect sizes were modest, so the following matching effects yielded only small improvements in drinking outcomes. TSF was more effective for outpatient clients without additional psychopathology, for outpatients with high social support for continued drinking, and for aftercare clients high in alcohol dependence. MET was more effective for outpatients high in anger. CBT was more effective for aftercare clients low in alcohol dependence. Thus, treatment matching studies have not shown consistent results regarding the efficacy of CBT for specific client types.

Meta-Analyses of Alcoholism Treatment Outcome Studies

In the past decade, a number of meta-analyses have compared the outcomes of various categories of alcoholism treatment. Among three independent meta-analyses, coping skills training interventions were ranked either 1 (Holder, Longabaugh, Miller, & Rubonis, 1991) or 2 (Miller et al., 1995; Finney & Monahan, 1996) among alcoholism treatments, based on evidence of effectiveness.

In addition to their review of studies of mediating mechanisms described earlier, Morgenstern and Longabaugh (2000) also conducted a box-score analysis focused on studies of CBT skills training approaches. They found that when added to another treatment, CBT did enhance treatment effectiveness, but that as a stand-alone treatment or aftercare, CBT was not superior to alternative treatments. The more potent the alternative to which CBT was compared, the less likely it was found to be more effective than the control treatment: It was superior to no-treatment controls and to some kinds of treatments, but it was no more effective than robust treatments.

A treatment approach that is closely related to coping skills training, relapse prevention (RP; Marlatt & Gordon, 1985), incorporates many interpersonal and intrapersonal coping skills training elements, in order to enhance clients' ability to respond effectively to trigger situations that are most likely to arouse cravings to drink or to initiate a relapse to actual drinking. A meta-analysis by Irvin, Bowers, Dunn, and Wang (1999) indicated that RP has its primary impact on psychosocial functioning, with less effect on substance use outcomes. Carroll's (1996) review of RP-oriented studies found that RP demonstrated efficacy for substance use outcomes when compared to no-treatment controls or to some alternative treatments (such as sobriety education or supportive therapy), but when compared to other alternative treatments (such as problem-solving training), it was comparable in effects. The review also concluded that RP is effective for sustaining the effects of treatment and reducing the severity of subsequent relapses, but these benefits diminish with increasing time after treatment.

To conclude this review of outcome research, coping skills treatment for alcoholism has been extensively studied in randomized controlled clinical trials. Generally, results either favor coping skills training as a treatment adjunct or find it to be equivalent to some robust active treatments. Significant results were more likely to be found with approaches that used interpersonal skills training. Some treatment matching studies suggest that coping skills treatment is more effective than interactional therapy with more impaired clients, but this has not been a consistent finding, and one matching study indicated that interpersonal coping skills training may be useful for a broader range of clients than is the intrapersonal approach. Taken together, the accumulated evidence suggests that coping skills training deserves a solid place in the repertoire of clinicians who work with alcoholic clients.

EVIDENCE BASE FOR CUE EXPOSURE TREATMENT APPROACHES

CET is a treatment method that can be applied with either an alcohol abstinence or moderate drinking treatment goal.

Moderation-Oriented Cue Exposure Studies

The early evidence for the potential benefit of CET approaches came from a series of case studies in England that used priming dose(s) of beverage alcohol as cues. The cases generally involved alcoholics with a treatment goal of moderate drinking, and the methods generally involved having the alcoholics drink a moderate amount and then practice resisting any further drinking. Typically, the clients were asked to sniff, then taste, then drink one to four 1-ounce drinks of liquor and then to try not to drink any more. Unlike the idea of exposure with response prevention, they were all told they could drink more if they could not resist. Most of these cases reported good outcomes, such as no drinking-related absences from work (Pickens, Bigelow, & Griffiths, 1973), greatly reduced number of heavy drinking days (Hodgson & Rankin, 1976; Rankin, 1982), or complete abstinence during a 9-month follow-up (Blakey & Baker, 1980).

In recent years, there have been a few larger scale controlled studies of CET using randomized or sequential assignment to treatments with drinking outcome data collected during the follow-up period. The first two studies were conducted in England. One randomized controlled study enrolled 42 nondependent problem drinkers interested in learning moderate drinking (Sitharthan, Sitharthan, Hough, & Kavanaugh, 1997). Those assigned to CET consumed two or three standard drinks, then tried to resist drinking while they sniffed another drink. Over the next 6 months, those who received CET drank on fewer days and consumed fewer drinks per occasion than those who were taught skills for moderate drinking. A second randomized controlled study assigned 91 alcoholics to either moderation-oriented cue exposure or behavioral self-control training without cue exposure (Heather et al., 2000). Both treatments worked equally well in reducing drinking during the 6-month follow-up period.

Abstinence-Oriented Cue Exposure Studies

A controlled study in England used an abstinence-oriented approach with hospitalized alcoholics (Drummond & Glautier, 1994). In CET, the client simply handled a drink for 40 minutes/day for 10 days. A 6-month follow-up of 32 clients showed that those receiving CET took significantly longer before resuming heavy drinking than did the clients receiving relaxation training.

A randomized controlled study in America with alcohol-dependent clients in an abstinence-oriented hospital program compared six sessions of CET, as described in Chapter 4, to no additional treatment (Monti et al., 1993). Participants were taught the urge-specific coping skills described in Chapter 4, plus urge reduction imagery (Marlatt & Gordon, 1985), cognitive mastery statements, and imagery of being in pleasant environments. For the first 3 months of follow-up, the 32 clients did equally well, but in the next 3 months, those in CET had a higher incidence of continuous abstinence, a higher number of abstinent days, and tended to have fewer drinks per day than the comparison clients. Measures of treatment process revealed that those who received CET had decreased urge to drink more during treatment than did the comparison clients. Also, clients in CET were more likely to use two of the coping strategies during the follow-up period: thinking about positive and negative consequences of use. More frequent use of these strategies was correlated with less drinking during the follow-up.

Next, a larger study compared CET (as described in Chapter 4) to relaxation and meditation while also comparing the interpersonal skills training (described in Chapter 2), called communication skills training (CST), to sobriety education. All study treatments were offered as treatment adjuncts for 100 alcohol-dependent clients from three residential or day treatment sites (Rohsenow et al., 2001). The effects of the CST intervention were described in a previous section of this chapter. During the first 6 months after discharge from treatment, those in CET had significantly fewer heavy drinking days (about 4% of days) than those in the comparison treatment (about 7% of days). During the next 6 months, among those who drank at all, those in CET drank on fewer days (15% of days) than those in the comparison condition (25% of days), and those who received both CET and CST drank significantly less (about 6 drinks on drinking days) than did those who received either CST alone or CET alone (about 11 to 13 drinks on drinking days).

Some data were also obtained in this study about processes that mediated the effects of treatment on drinking outcomes. First, CET did not seem to work by reducing reactions to alcohol beverage cues, at least not in a laboratory situation. Second, those who received CET showed more reductions in urge to drink in an assessment of high-risk situations than did comparison clients. Third, at each follow-up interview, clients were asked about strategies they had used to stay abstinent when they experienced an urge to drink. Those who received CET used more of the strategies that they had been taught than did those in the comparison condition, and use of the five strategies described in Chapter 4 was predictive of a lower quantity and frequency of drinking at the 6- and 12-month interviews. Therefore, the form of CET described in this book appears to have its beneficial effects primarily by allowing clients to practice urge-specific coping skills while experiencing strong urges as a result either of beverage exposure or imagining a high-risk situation.

Abstinence-Oriented Cue Exposure Plus Interpersonal Skills Training

One additional study treated alcohol-dependent clients in a day treatment program either with CET and CST combined, or with a comparison treatment, meditation–relaxation, and sobriety education combined, all treatments conducted in group format (Monti et al., 2001). After a week or so in day treatment, clients randomly received 12 weeks of either naltrexone or a placebo along with outpatient visits. The results for naltrexone are described later in this chapter. During the first 3 months after leaving day treatment, alcoholics in both the behavioral treatment conditions did equally well, with only 40% drinking at all, and only 30% having a heavy drinking day. From 4 to 12 months, those who received CET and CST were significantly less likely to have any heavy drinking day than those in the comparison treatments, and had fewer heavy drinking days. Basically, those who received CET and CST maintained their initial treatment successes, whereas those in the comparison treatments drank more during the 12 months of follow-up. Only four to five sessions of CET and CST were given to each client, yet this brief treatment had lasting effects, even when added to an already rich treatment program. Therefore, this brief approach may be particularly beneficial in the context of managed care.

Treatment process measures showed that clients who received CET and CST improved more in their confidence that they could cope with a set of high-risk situations without drinking (self-efficacy), and this improved self-efficacy predicted lower drinking rates at 3, 6, and 12 months. Clients who received CET and CST also reported lower urge to drink in a posttreatment laboratory assessment of their reactions to alcohol, and lower urge to drink in this assessment predicted less drinking during the 6- and 12-month follow-ups. Finally, clients who received CET and CST reported using more urge-specific and general coping strategies during the follow-up, which in turn predicted less drinking at the 3-, 6-, and 12-month follow-ups.

In summary, the controlled trials of CET fairly consistently show beneficial effects of CET on treatment outcomes, both when used for moderation training, and when used in abstinence-oriented treatment. CET was found to improve outcomes when administered as pure exposure alone or in the approach combining cue exposure with coping skills training, as described in this book. The combined approach allows clients to practice coping with urges induced by beverages and other drinking triggers while in the safety of the therapist's office, and in this way may provide an advantage over pure exposure-based approaches.

IMPLICATIONS OF RECENT INNOVATIONS

A few exciting innovations developed in the last decade are worth mentioning. We describe some of these innovations and their implications for applying the skills training model.

Stages of Change: Implications for Skills Training

A model of the therapeutic change process has been developed that incorporates consideration of people's readiness to change their behavior when planning treatment interventions. This transtheoretical model of change (Prochaska & DiClemente, 1986; DiClemente, 1991) proposes that people with a problem behavior such as alcohol dependence can at any moment be more or less ready to change their behavior. If the client is not currently motivated to quit drinking, he/she may not pay attention to treatment material designed to help clients learn how to quit and stay off alcohol. The skills training approaches described in this book are essentially designed for people who are motivated for sobriety. Implications of this model for handling less motivated clients are presented in Chapter 6.

New Pharmacotherapies

For most of the past 30 years, the only pharmacotherapy specifically designed to treat alcoholism has been disulfiram (Antabuse™), which works by blocking part of the metabolism of alcohol, so that alcohol ingestion causes people to feel very uncomfortable. Although disulfiram is effective as a deterrent to drinking while people take it, it does not affect urge to drink, and when people want to return to drinking, they simply stop taking it. In a multisite study of 605 clients randomized to disulfiram or placebo, only 20% of clients continued taking the medication, and disulfiram worked no better than placebo in promoting abstinence or delaying relapse (Fuller et al., 1986). However, disulfiram works best when procedures are set up to have another person observe and reinforce the intake of the medication, and when coping skills training focused on RP is conducted in conjunction with it (Azrin, Sisson, Meyers, & Godley, 1982).

In the past decade, naltrexone (ReVia™) has been approved for use with alcoholics. Naltrexone is an opiate blocker that seems to work by decreasing the release of chemicals (such as dopamine) in the parts of the brain associated with the pleasurable effects of alcohol and other drugs (the mesolimbic system). In several studies, naltrexone was shown to decrease drinking among alcoholics during the 12 weeks they were prescribed and taking it (e.g., Volpicelli, Alterman, Hayashida, & O'Brien, 1992; O'Malley et al., 1992; Monti et al., 2001). Rather than being intended as the sole treatment, it was found to be more effective in reducing relapse for clients who also received RP training (O'Malley et al., 1992). One particular advantage of naltrexone is that it reduces urges to drink, as reported in daily ratings by outpatients (O'Malley et al., 1995; Monti et al., 2001) and when clients are confronted with the sight and smell of their favorite alcohol beverage (Monti et al., 1999), even after a single dose of naltrexone (Rohsenow, Monti, Hutchinson, et al., 2000). One drawback of naltrexone is that many clients are uninterested in taking it, and a great many do not stay on it for even the 12 weeks currently recommended. Compliance is lower among clients who experience side effects (especially fatigue or nausea), who have less of a belief that naltrexone is an effective medication, or who have comorbid drug abuse (Rohsenow, Colby, et al., 2000). A second drawback is that its beneficial effects dissipate within a few months after the course of naltrexone is completed.

Although naltrexone has not proven to be quite the magic bullet that some once hoped, it has nevertheless met with some clinical success and has enabled the development of a laboratory-based procedure to analyze the mechanism of action of this and other pharmacotherapies. The cue exposure paradigm through which naltrexone has demonstrated urge reduction (Monti et al., 1999) has the potential to bridge the gap between the laboratory and clinical trials (Monti, Rohsenow, & Hutchison, 2000) and may thus help in the development of more sophisticated pharmacotherapies in a relatively efficient manner.

Also of interest are some implications of combining naltrexone with skills training approaches. First, during skills training, therapists can bolster clients' compliance with the medication by helping them anticipate and more effectively manage the side effects, and by bolstering their belief that naltrexone is an effective medication (Rohsenow, Colby, et al., 2000). Second, naltrexone might be a good supplement to skills training, because it produces beneficial results during the early weeks of outpatient treatment, when skills training may still be underway and not yet having differential benefit, whereas skills training and CET may exert maximum benefit from 3 months to at least a year, when naltrexone is no longer having differential benefit.

One treatment consideration is the timing of when to start naltrexone treatment. Many clients have elevated liver function tests when first presenting for treatment and therefore may need to be excluded from naltrexone treatment initially, but waiting a week or so often allows clients' medical condition to improve to the point that they may be medically eligible for naltrexone. During the wait, skills training can be conducted intensively, until the client is eligible for naltrexone. However, if CET is to be conducted, naltrexone should be further delayed until the CET is completed. Because CET depends in part on eliciting urges and other reactions to the alcohol cues and drinking triggers, and naltrexone diminishes some of these reactions, it could prevent CET from being effective. Therefore, CET should be conducted prior to starting naltrexone treatment.

Acamprosate, a medication used with alcoholics in Europe, is a medication that we are likely to see approved for use in the United States within the next decade. Acamprosate affects the gamma-aminobutyric acid (GABA) receptors, a different mechanism of action than naltrexone or many psychotropic medications. In 10 out of 11 controlled treatment trials conducted in Europe, acamprosate resulted in more abstinence than did placebo, with the follow-up periods usually lasting at least a year (Anton et al., 1996). For example, among 272 alcoholics treated for 48 weeks in Germany, 43% of those on acamprosate were completely abstinent compared to 21% of those on placebo (Sass, Soyka, Mann, & Zieglgansberger, 1996). When acamprosate is approved, probably most of the same treatment considerations discussed for integrating naltrexone with skills training will apply with this new medication as well.

It is clear from this chapter that the treatment field has advanced quite impressively over the past decade. However, large numbers of alcohol-dependent people still need our help. Furthermore, the fact that alcohol has begun to impact the lives of young people negatively at ever greater rates (Johnston, O'Malley, & Bachman, 1999) suggests that effective treatment approaches will be needed as these youth enter treatment programs. It is our hope that the revised edition of *Treating Alcohol Dependence* will not only enjoy the same popularity as the earlier book among treatment providers and researchers, but that it will also stimulate new thinking on how to improve the treatment of persons plagued with alcohol problems.

TWO

General Treatment Considerations: Setting the Stage and Treatment Setting

Introduction   19

Setting the Stage   20

Partial Hospital and Day Treatment Considerations   30

Outpatient and Aftercare Considerations   31

Individual Treatment Considerations   39

INTRODUCTION

A set of process and procedural issues have emerged from our clinical work that we feel are as important to ensuring the effectiveness of the coping skills training program as the basic elements to be presented in Chapters 3 and 4. In this chapter, we discuss these treatment process issues as they pertain to conducting coping skills training group and individual treatment with alcoholics. Many of these issues are not unique to our program with alcoholics (cf. Vannicelli, 1992). Indeed, we have discussed similar issues pertaining to treatment of other psychiatric populations (e.g., Monti, Corriveau, & Curran, 1982b; Monti & Kolko, 1985), as have other authors (e.g., Upper & Ross, 1985). Yet there are some important key elements in working with alcoholics, and these receive particular emphasis here.

In the context of behavioral skills training groups, "process" can have a somewhat different meaning than it does in other types of group psychotherapy. Behavioral skills training groups are not a process of exploration of whatever issues come up in the here and now, nor are they a didactic lecture series. Because the goal of such a group is to educate clients rather than to explore underlying psychodynamic conflicts, many of the process

19

comments in this chapter pertain to pragmatic issues of how to ensure the learning and practice of new behaviors. This requires more than the group's listening attentively to a didactic lecture. It is an engaging series of interactions between therapists and group members, and among group members themselves—one that is (we hope) relevant and even enjoyable.

A balance must be struck between allowing for group autonomy and ensuring that specific skills are taught and practiced. All group members must get a chance to build their actual skills during role plays and to receive constructive feedback, using relevant (client-centered) problems. As Bandura (1977) points out, active participation, modeling, and practice with positive, corrective feedback are the most effective ways to modify self-efficacy expectations and create long-lasting behavior change.

In this cognitive-behavioral approach, many of the basic rules for conducting psychotherapy groups apply. Therapists must use many traditional group therapy skills (e.g., establishing rapport, limit setting, empathy), while at the same time functioning as active trainers and role models for the group.

A number of unique problems are likely to arise in dealing with groups of alcoholic clients. An excellent review of these, and some suggested responses to them, is provided by Vannicelli (1992). Although those suggestions are based on a dynamic interactional model of group therapy (Yalom, 1974; Yalom, Block, Bond, Zimmerman, & Qualls, 1978), descriptions of potential problems and suggested behavioral interventions have proven helpful to our group leaders.

This chapter consists of several parts. First, we present general treatment process issues that are important to set the stage for conducting skills training, including topics such as therapist training, cotherapist teams, developing the rationale and techniques for role playing, between-session (homework) assignments, motivational issues, and incorporating significant others (e.g., family members) into the treatment groups. The second section deals with treatment process/procedural issues that are especially relevant to partial hospital or day treatment settings, including topics such as integrating coping skills training with other treatment modalities, communication among staff members, neuropsychological factors that may be present after recent detoxification, and dealing with severe psychopathology. The third section presents considerations for conducting coping skills training with outpatients and deals with issues such as the advantages of outpatient treatment, transition from partial hospital to outpatient treatment, group ground rules, the order of topics, attrition, and termination. In a final section, we consider issues pertinent to conducting our program as individual therapy in a one-on-one situation.

SETTING THE STAGE

Responsibility for Change

Some have argued that if one accepts as fact that addictive behaviors are learned, then it is equivalent to "blaming the victim" (Sontag, 1978). According to this line of reasoning, behavior theorists in effect hold addicted individuals personally responsible for having acquired and continuing in their self-destructive behavior patterns. However, this perspective is based on the false assumption that individuals are somehow to be held responsible for their earlier learning experiences. Marlatt (1985c) counters this assumption:

Behavioral theorists define addiction as a powerful habit pattern, an acquired vicious cycle of self-destructive behavior that is locked in by the collective effects of classical conditioning (acquired tolerance mediated in part by classically conditioned compensatory responses to the deleterious effects of the addictive substance), and operant reinforcement (both the positive reinforcement of the high of the drug rush and the negative reinforcement associated with drug use as a means of escaping or avoiding dysphoric physical and/or mental states—including those associated with the negative aftereffects of prior drug use). In terms of conditioning factors alone, an individual who acquires an addictive habit is no more to be held responsible for this behavior than one of Pavlov's dogs would be held responsible for salivating at the sound of a ringing bell. In addition to classical and operant conditioning factors, human drug use is also determined to a large extent by acquired expectancies and beliefs about drugs as an antidote to stress and anxiety. Social learning and modeling factors (observational learning) also exert a strong influence (e.g., drug use in the family and peer environment, along with the pervasive portrayal of drug use in advertising and the media). Just because a behavioral problem can be described as a learned habit pattern does not imply that the person is to be held responsible for the acquisition of the habit, nor that the individual is capable of exercising voluntary control over the behavior. (p. 11)

Although the individual may not be responsible for acquiring the addiction, he/she needs to take active responsibility for participating in treatment. Social learning theory-based *treatment* for alcohol abuse and dependence requires active participation by the individual client, as well as his/her assumption of responsibility for learning the necessary skills to prevent future abuse. Through active participation in a training program in which new skills and cognitive strategies are acquired, an individual's maladaptive habits can be replaced with healthy behaviors regulated by cognitive processes involving awareness and responsible planning.

The interested reader is referred to Brickman et al. (1982) for an extensive discussion of the distinction between attribution of responsibility for the development of a problem and attribution of responsibility for a solution. Therapists should be prepared to discuss this distinction. They can empathize with the clients over their difficult history and then instill hope for the future by suggesting that it is never too late to learn how to take better care of oneself. This can be accomplished by learning self-management and coping skills that were lost or never learned adequately heretofore.

Therapist Training

As is the case for all types of therapy, there is no substitute for a well-trained therapist. Therapists must be experienced in psychotherapy skills as well as behavioral principles. In addition, they must have good interpersonal skills and be familiar with the training materials, so as to impart skills successfully and serve as credible models. They must be willing to play a very active role in this type of *directive* group and individual therapy.

A master's degree in a mental health discipline (e.g., counseling, psychiatric nursing, psychology), is generally considered as "entry level" for our therapists, although we occasionally employ bachelor's-level individuals as cotherapists. We also feel that some clinical experience in treating alcoholics is just as important as academic degrees. Usually, 1 year of experience is the minimum that is acceptable.

Therapist training consists of several stages. In the first stage, we encourage trainees to review the entire training program (Chapters 2, 3, 4, and 5 of this volume). In addition, we assign several key review papers as general background material. Chapter 1 provides an overview of material we present to our trainees. Next, the trainees frequently observe sessions of an ongoing treatment through a one-way mirror. A doctoral-level therapist supervisor is usually present, along with the therapist trainee observing the group, enabling the supervisor to point out particular aspects of the treatment as they occur. The trainee is encouraged to ask questions as they arise. Following each session, the trainee meets with the supervisor and the therapist or cotherapists to debrief for 10–15 minutes. In the third stage, after a therapist trainee has observed one full treatment cycle, he/she usually participates in a group as a role-play partner or substitute therapist, or in cue exposure treatment as the more active partner. Feedback is provided after each session in this "hands-on" forum. In the last stage of training for groups, the trainee is paired with an experienced therapist to form a cotherapy team. In addition to postsession debriefings, 1 hour of supervision per week is provided by the supervisor.

When treatment is observed through a one-way mirror in the first treatment session, a therapist explains who will be observing and why. To desensitize clients and to enhance trust and direct communication between therapists and clients, a therapist invites the supervisor and trainee(s) into the treatment room for a moment to be introduced, and the client or group members are encouraged to ask questions. Our experience suggests that several minutes invested in this way during the first session usually satisfy any concerns that clients might have about being observed.

Cotherapist Teams

Except during cue exposure treatment, our therapy program is usually led by cotherapist teams. We prefer that a male and a female team up together, regardless of the composition of the group, to ensure that models of both sexes are available. If there are no women in a particular group, as was often the case on our alcohol treatment wards at the Veterans Affairs Medical Centers, then the presence of a female cotherapist is especially important to provide adequate modeling. However, given the economic constraints at many treatment centers, these approaches can certainly be conducted by one therapist alone.

If cotherapists are available, each of the therapists is encouraged to assume either a "content" or a "process" role for each session. The "content" therapist is responsible for ensuring that the necessary material for a particular session is adequately covered. The "process" therapist is responsible for attending to and responding to process issues as they emerge during the session. For example, if one therapist is so involved in describing skills that he/she does not pick up on the fact that group members are bored and not paying attention, then the process therapist may interrupt by suggesting a relevant example, so as to stimulate more members to tune in. The therapists should shift process and content roles in alternate sessions to prevent role stereotyping.

Good communication and cooperation between cotherapists are important; they not only affect the tone of the session but also provide ongoing modeling for group members (e.g., how to disagree agreeably, how to listen, how to use nonverbal behaviors). Some cotherapists "click" at the outset and spontaneously work well together. Others require more effort to work together. Elements to remain aware of in doing effective cotherapy include the following:

1. Knowing and accepting each other's role in a particular session (e.g., content or process).

2. Knowing each other's strengths and weaknesses with respect to role-playing and communication skills.

3. Taking equal responsibility for various procedures across sessions, such as introducing new topics, providing feedback after role-play exercises, assigning practice exercises, being empathetic and supportive, encouraging less verbal clients to become more actively involved in the group, and so on.

4. Looking at, tracking, and asking each other for input at various points throughout the session. The cotherapists should follow up on each other's comments and allow each other "room" to pursue a point.

5. Therapists should not hesitate to articulate their differences of opinion. This provides an excellent opportunity to model the negotiation of compromises.

Guidelines for Therapists

Prior to each treatment session, therapists are encouraged to reread relevant sections of the manual. To ensure that the main points of each session are covered, we recommend bringing in an outline of the points. To standardize the delivery of this material, we have developed and routinely use large poster boards that summarize the Skill Guidelines for each session. Alternatively, the points can be made on a blackboard, which better allows individual examples to be added within the session.

Even though use of a manual increases the likelihood that all relevant material will be covered, this should not lead to reading to clients from the text verbatim. As long as the major points are covered, a natural, free-flowing presentation style is preferred. It is crucial that clients not get the message that the therapists' agenda of adhering strictly to the manual is more important than the issues and concerns that constitute their personal agendas.

Indeed, if clients are not routinely involved and encouraged to provide their own material as examples, we have found that the groups become boring and the energy level for learning drops off dramatically. Therapists may experience burnout as a result. If a group becomes boring, it may be a sign of a burned out therapist, because therapists must maintain a high level of energy and enthusiasm at all times. Effective reinforcement of clients for their active participation can help prevent burnout on the part of both clients and therapists.

The Rationale and Skill Guidelines sections of each session in Chapters 3 and 4 are intended to provide therapists with adequate background information to guide discussion of each topic. Although the topics covered usually generate group discussion that is meaningful, the discussion must be shaped by the therapists to prevent it from shifting focus onto other clinical issues (e.g., lengthy accounts of personal material). Because the treatment session can pass very quickly, it is important that the therapists keep the presentation of the Rationale and Skill Guidelines brief, to allow the majority of time for the role plays, feedback, and group discussion of clients' experiences in practicing the skills. Discussion must be even briefer in cue exposure treatment (CET), because most of the session must involve the active exposure to cues.

As in other clinical work, appropriate self-disclosure and humor can be helpful clinical tools. As long as proper clinical judgment regarding timing and content is exercised, it can be helpful if therapists share with the group some of their own dilemmas and coping strategies. This demonstrates that group members are not alone in their efforts to cope with problem situations.

One self-disclosure issue likely to come up at the beginning of therapy for alcoholics is the question regarding the drinking practices of the therapists (Vannicelli, 1982). Therapists differ as to whether or not to answer this question directly; however, we agree with Vannicelli that the real concern being expressed is "Will you, therapist, be able to understand me, and can I get the kind of help here that I need?" (p. 21). Thus, although we leave the specific answer to this question up to our therapists' judgment and individual therapeutic styles, we do encourage them to acknowledge to the client(s) asking the question that they hear the underlying message. How this question is handled can be important, because many clients are only familiar with Alcoholics Anonymous (AA) or other groups led by counselors who are themselves recovering alcoholics. Acknowledgment of the clients' underlying concern, coupled with an invitation to judge the value of this program for themselves, usually is adequate.

A related concern involves alcoholics' expectations as to what the skill training approach is all about. Many alcoholics are familiar with AA groups, which are highly structured, or with traditional psychotherapy groups, where an attempt is made to explore feelings and resolve conflicts. Although clients are informed that the exploration of feelings and resolution of conflicts can occur in the sessions, the emphasis is on skills training and behavioral or mental rehearsal. It is important also to note that our approach is entirely compatible with that of AA. To this end, we recommend that our therapists familiarize themselves with the similarities and differences between an AA approach and a behavioral approach to treatment (McCrady & Miller, 1993), so that they are prepared to clarify questions that clients might have. (See the "Outpatient and Aftercare Considerations" section of this chapter for further information on how to prepare clients for coping skills treatment.)

Guidelines for Behavior Rehearsal Role Plays

Behavior rehearsal is the main strategy by which group members acquire new skills in the interpersonal and intrapersonal approaches in Chapter 3 and 4, and imaginal rehearsal of behaviors is the main method of acquiring skills in CET in Chapter 5. Each session provides a "safe haven," where members can practice and improve their skills prior to taking the risk of trying them out in the real world. This safe haven is particularly important when learning to cope with real urges to drink in CET. Although some group discussion during the introduction to each new skill is useful, therapists should discourage lengthy discussion about problem situations, and instead should focus on setting up and processing role plays or cue exposure situations.

It is normal for group members (and therapists!) to feel a bit uncomfortable or embarrassed at first about role playing in front of the rest of the group. Therapists should acknowledge that this is a normal reaction, and that behavior rehearsal becomes easier after a few experiences with it. After a while, participants are able to "get into" a scene more realistically and to focus on their role in it.

Resistance to role playing can take subtle forms, such as focusing on other issues or asking many questions. It may be very tempting to become sidetracked into exploring other issues raised by resistant individuals in the group. Therapists can acknowledge that they also feel uncomfortable role playing in front of a group of strangers; they may have to take the lead and demonstrate the first role plays. Often, if a therapist simply starts a role-played scenario with a client, the client will respond in role.

Therapists should encourage clients to generate and describe personally relevant scenes that are initially of only moderate difficulty. As clients demonstrate ability to handle these situations effectively, they should be encouraged to generate and practice more difficult ones. An adequate description of a scene includes specifying where it takes place, the primary problems/goals, whom the role-play partner should portray (boss, stranger, child, spouse, date, etc.), and relevant behaviors of the person portrayed so that the partner can act accordingly. See Tip Sheet for questions that can elicit this information.

The following strategies are useful in helping group members to generate scenes:

1. Recall a situation in the recent past in which use of the new skill being taught would have been desirable (e.g., a client wanted to start a conversation but couldn't; another yelled at a neighbor about an unleashed dog tearing up the garden; still another wanted to express positive feelings toward his/her spouse but couldn't without drinking first).

2. Anticipate a difficult situation that may arise in the near future that calls for use of the new skill (e.g., a client's apartment has been cold this winter and he/she wants to ask the building owner to raise the setting on the thermostat; another client is going to a retirement party this weekend and will be offered alcoholic drinks).

3. The group leader can suggest an appropriate situation based on his/her knowledge of a group member's recent circumstances (e.g., "I know you've been wanting to get a sponsor at AA but have been shy about approaching someone about it. How about setting up a scene involving the end of an AA meeting at which the person you'd like as a sponsor is present? Where might he/she be standing? In a group of people? Alone at the coffee table?")

4. A group leader can use self-disclosure about a situation in which he/she has difficulty to aid clients in thinking about situations from their own lives. For example, a therapist might say, "A person I live with always leaves the top off the toothpaste. It's certainly not a major problem, but it does bother me, and if I don't speak up about it, I find that I start to get more irritated about it every day, until I finally get real angry at him/her. Then, we have an argument that could easily have been avoided if I'd just spoken up sooner and said it differently. What kinds of 'little' things like this do you stew over until you get upset, rather than speaking up in the first place?"

5. The therapists can create a hypothetical situation for role playing. This approach should only be employed in the rare instances when the other strategies are insufficient.

It is essential that each role play be processed in a way that makes it a productive and encouraging learning experience for the participants. It is an opportunity for participants to receive social praise/recognition for practice and improvement, as well as constructive criticism about the less effective elements of their behavior. During this portion of the session, the therapists' primary goals are first to shape and reinforce successive approximations to more effective skills and then to identify specific problems with skills implementation.

Immediately after every role play, therapists should reinforce both role-play partners for participating, then elicit feedback from all who are present:

1. Ask both partners to give their reactions to the performance (e.g., How does the protagonist feel about the way he/she handled the situation? What effect did the interaction have on the partner?).

2. Ask other group members to offer comments. Respond to those comments in a manner that encourages group members to focus on relevant issues in a constructive fashion. Initially, until therapists have modeled giving constructive criticism once or twice, they might solicit only positive feedback from group members (e.g., "What was good about the way John handled that situation?"). To the extent that group members offer supportive feedback and constructive criticism, they provide each other with a very valuable source of encouragement and ideas.

3. The therapists then offer their own comments about the role play. As already emphasized, these comments should be both supportive/reinforcing and constructively critical. If there are several deficiencies in a role-play performance, the therapists should choose only one or two to work on at a time. Both positive and negative feedback should focus on *specific* aspects of the person's behavior, because global evaluations do not pinpoint what was particularly effective or ineffective. Finally, the therapists should refrain from being unnecessarily effusive, so that the value of the positive feedback is not undermined.

Therapists may also have the role-play partners repeat a scene to give the protagonist an opportunity to try out the feedback they received the first time around. However, given the time limitations of the session, therapists will need to be attentive to striking a reasonable balance between doing repeat role plays and moving on to a new scene to give other group members a chance to practice. A Tip Sheet provides a summary list of Behavior Rehearsal Role-Play Guidelines.

"Role reversal" is a role-play strategy in which the therapist (or a skillful group member) models use of the new skill, with the client playing the role of the target person (e.g., spouse, employer, neighbor). This strategy is particularly useful if a client is having difficulty using a skill or is pessimistic about the effectiveness of a suggested communication approach. By playing the "other," he/she has an opportunity to observe and to experience firsthand the effects of the suggested skill.

Review Sessions

Review sessions can be scheduled every fourth or fifth session. The primary reason for frequent reviews is to foster practice and retention of newly learned material, despite the cognitive impairment that often occurs early in alcoholics' recovery. Recent sessions are reviewed in detail, including skills guidelines and role playing. Clients are asked to discuss their experience in applying these new skills to their daily lives, and problems they may have encountered in doing so. The group brainstorms solutions to problems that have been encountered, and members try role playing the solutions arrived at by this process. During the review sessions that occur later in the program, recent sessions are not only reviewed but also some brief review of earlier sessions is provided.

Review is not entirely confined to specified review sessions. During the initial portion of every session, when clients discuss problems they encounter in their daily lives, the therapists have an opportunity to review previously taught skills that may be applied to resolve the problems. This may involve review of specific skills guidelines, as well as role playing those skills.

Practice Exercises Outside of Sessions (Homework)

Homework is a powerful adjunct to treatment, utilizing real-life situations for out-of-group practice. This offers the distinct advantage of practice in actual problem situations, enhancing the likelihood that these behaviors will be repeated in similar situations (generalization). A preplanned homework exercise has been designed for every session of our interpersonal and intrapersonal skills approaches. (As part of CET, we strongly discourage clients from deliberately exposing themselves to cues on their own, although we encourage their use of the coping strategies if drinking triggers occur unexpectedly.) Most homework assignments require that the client try in a real-life situation what he/she has already role-played in the group session. The homework assignment may also require that the client record facts concerning the setting, his/her behavior, the response it evoked, and an evaluation of the adequacy of his/her performance. Homework exercises can be modified to fit the specific details of individual situations more closely, and extra homework assignments are sometimes given to help clients cope with problem situations they have encountered.

It should be pointed out that although outpatient and partial hospital settings are perhaps more conducive to multiple opportunities for homework practice, the residential setting does provide some opportunities as well. Clients in residential settings should be encouraged to practice assignments with visitors and/or other patients on their units, or when on passes. If no other individuals are available for practice, clients should be encouraged to approach members of the treatment staff as role-play partners. The urge coping skills learned in CET can also be practiced in the residential setting as interactions or discussions elicit urges.

Compliance with homework is often a problem in behavior therapy in general, and these groups are no exception. A number of steps are taken to foster compliance. The assignments are referred to as "Practice Exercises" to avoid the negative connotations often associated with the term "homework." When giving each assignment, the therapists provide a rationale and description of the assignment. They ask the group members what problems they can foresee in completing the assignment, and discuss ways to overcome these obstacles. Clients are asked to identify a specific time that can be set aside to work on the homework assignment. Therapists review the preceding session's homework exercises at the beginning of each session, making an effort to praise all approximations to compliance with the assignment. Although problems that clients have with the exercises should certainly be discussed, the main emphasis is on reinforcing the positive aspects of performance. For those who did not do an assignment, group suggestions are solicited as to what might be done to ensure compliance with the next assignment.

When critiquing role plays and homework assignments, it should be noted and communicated to clients (depending on their level of functioning) that "coping models" may have a greater impact on changing behavior than do "mastery models."

Dealing with Less Motivated Clients

In the past decade, increased attention has been paid to the effect of differing levels of motivation for change on receptiveness to treatment (see Miller & Rollnick, 2002, for a full discussion of this topic). Clients may have been required by someone else to attend substance abuse treatment but may not have intrinsic motivation to change their substance use (precontemplation stage), may have been thinking about changing their substance use someday but not be ready to change at this time (contemplation stage), may be determined to cut down or quit their substance of abuse (preparation stage), may have recently quit drinking or using (action stage), or may have been sober for more than 6 months (maintenance stage) but then experienced a slip that brought them into treatment.

Clients may shift between these stages on a day-to-day or minute-by-minute basis as their motivational level waxes and wanes. If treatments are designed for clients who have decided to change, and want to learn how to change, those who have not yet decided to make a change might think these approaches are irrelevant to their needs and may consequently fail to pay attention. Such motivational issues have several implications for the skills training approaches described herein, because they are oriented primarily toward clients in the determination, action, and maintenance stages.

For example, clients who are precontemplators or even contemplators might initially benefit from one to three sessions of motivational interviewing designed to enhance their readiness to change. The methods in the book by Miller and Rollnick (2002) are best for this approach. In our experience, several strategies have been effective with the less motivated clients. First, we roll with resistance and avoid arguing, as Miller and Rollnick (2002) teach. Instead, we suggest that most of the interpersonal and intrapersonal skills that will be taught are useful in dealing with numerous situations in clients' lives, whether substances are involved or not. In this way, clients may learn the skills for various reasons and will then have them available for use in drinking as well as other situations after treatment. Second, other clients in the groups generally effectively provide encouragement and increase the motivational level of initially resistant clients within a relatively short period of time. Third, the CET approach (as described in Chapter 5) has been effective at breaking through clients' resistance in many cases. Clients who were sure that they had no urges to drink have often been surprised by the strong urges produced by the cues and have then become considerably more receptive to treatment.

Clearly, attention to clients' motivational level from the start, and throughout the treatment process, with appropriate accommodation of treatment according to their motivation at a particular time, is likely to result in the most effective intervention.

Coping Skills Training with Significant Others Included

There is a growing literature on the role of family interaction and marital communication difficulties in the maintenance of alcohol abuse. Maladaptive patterns of communication, lack of intimacy, and control struggles can be precipitants of drinking (Epstein & McCrady, 1998). Including significant others in skills treatment can greatly enhance the likelihood of recovery, and the maintenance and generalization of change (Monti & Kolko, 1985). However, it should be noted that the approach in Chapter 3 is equally effective with or without family member inclusion (Monti et al., 1990).

Several practical hurdles must be overcome in recruiting and retaining significant others in treatment. In one of our residential settings, a requirement for admission is to have at least one significant, nonalcoholic member of a client's social network available to participate in treatment. In practice, most alcoholics are able to come up with someone to satisfy this admission criterion. If a program's leaders are not willing or able to set such a stringent contingency on treatment, it may be difficult to encourage some clients to identify persons willing to participate fully.

Another common problem is scheduling. Ideally, having family groups meet two or three times per week is desirable, but most significant others cannot make such a large time commitment. We found that an extended (2-hour) group session held once per week for several weeks is an acceptable compromise.

The emphasis in these family sessions should be placed on interpersonal skills training topics (i.e., the material in Chapter 3). Individually focused cognitive and intrapersonal exercises can be provided to the alcoholics in separate sessions. Some couples may also need behavioral couple treatment (O'Farrell & Fals-Stewart, 2000). Group size, when family members participate, should be limited to 6 or 8 clients at most (i.e., 12–16 group members total).

A group coping skills training program can be beneficial to both clients and significant others for reducing dysfunctional interactions, but it does not necessarily result in all the changes in functioning that would be the goal of family systems treatment (Steinglass, Bennett, Wolin, & Reiss, 1987). Nevertheless, the basic set of communication skills described in this book, directed at client and spouse behaviors, can be useful for changing interactions that could otherwise lead to relapse.

As an illustration, a spouse may challenge/criticize an alcoholic in a suspicious manner that, although intended to prevent drinking, may actually exacerbate the likelihood of drinking. The client and spouse can be taught directly, in role plays with each other, how to give and receive criticism in a more adaptive fashion. If the role play and feedback improve communication and reduce misunderstanding, then maintenance of sobriety is more likely.

Occasionally the relationship between a significant other and the alcoholic is so conflicted that effective role playing cannot take place initially. In these circumstances, we have found it helpful to first have the therapists role-play the skills in question. Following this, the significant other is paired with one therapist and the scenario is repeated, followed by feedback from group members. Next, the alcoholic will role-play with the other therapist. Finally, the alcoholic will be paired with his/her significant other. By this time, after receiving feedback on several role plays, the pair may be better equipped to engage in effective role playing together.

In couples with a great deal of marital distress, it is best not to try to deal with all of the complex marital and perhaps even sexual dysfunction issues in the group. It is sometimes useful to limit the skills training focus to more basic, "safe" skills (i.e., giving and receiving compliments, criticism, assertiveness, nonverbal behavior), at least early on, and to refer them to adjunctive couple therapy.

A more difficult but essential next step is to explore communication concerning drinking behaviors and triggers of drinking. Such an exploration may lead to more deep-seated marital conflicts over trust, anger, intimacy, abandonment, dependence, and narcissistic needs. Sometimes these issues can be dealt with briefly in the group, but they tend to require large amounts of time and, consequently, the skills training materials may not get covered. Therapists need to bring the focus back to the specific observable behaviors that appear to be functionally related to drinking or poor communication skills. If it is obvious that more severe individual deficits (e.g., personality disorders) or severe marital distress exist, then the therapists should educate the clients (and the group) about the utility of other forms of psychotherapy or marital/family therapy.

PARTIAL HOSPITAL AND DAY TREATMENT CONSIDERATIONS

Treatment Goals

The relative "safety" offered by the partial hospital or day treatment setting as opposed to less intense settings allows therapists to elicit the emotions associated with clients' high-risk situations and provide enough support to minimize the risks to current sobriety. Given the frequency and intensity of treatment in a partial hospital setting, therapists quickly learn the existing strengths and weaknesses of group members. This knowledge may enable them to accelerate the intensity of training and thus maximize learning in a safe environment. Clients are taught appropriate coping skills, so that they can deal effectively with these situations without drinking. Cue exposure is ideally done in these settings (early in the day) to allow urges to dissipate after the CET session in safety, or to be processed in later treatment interactions.

Menu of Topics

Although we had originally recommended a sequence of topics that progresses from the easier and more concrete to the more difficult and complex, the advent of managed care has necessitated more flexibility, including entering clients into ongoing groups on a "rolling admissions" basis. This can be successfully accomplished by meeting with clients individually for a session or two to "bring them up to speed." Such accommodation is particularly important for those who may be experiencing residual cognitive impairment from alcohol detoxification.

The topics in each chapter have been designed to follow a 3- to 5-day detoxification period. When medications are used during detoxification, additional time may be required before alcoholics function at a cognitive level at which they can incorporate the skills presented in our program.

Our partial hospital sessions are typically 50–60 minutes long. They can be scheduled either daily or twice daily, depending on the length of the program. Because homework assignments are an important component of our treatment program, we recommend that two sessions per day be scheduled only when absolutely necessary. The exception is that CET in the morning followed by interpersonal or intrapersonal skills training either in the next hour or later, can be useful. Therapists may modify the topics or eliminate some sessions according to the needs of particular populations and programs.

Concurrent Treatments

Our program was designed to be integrated with other partial hospital treatment components, including alcohol education, occupational therapy, individual counseling, involvement in AA, and ongoing family groups. Because these other components may be derived from different theoretical schools, it is important to begin by presenting the rationale for the coping skills approach. We urge our therapists to stress the complementary aspects of coping skills training and CET as they relate to the contrasting treatment approaches. We have found it helpful to discuss topics such as how craving and relapse are linked to certain situations, moods, or thoughts; how a coping skills/social learning approach adds another dimension to understanding alcohol dependence; and the importance of assuming responsibility for one's recovery. Following Marlatt (1985c), one example that we have found helpful in clarifying the latter issue is the case of diabetes. If one takes insulin, watches his/her diet, and exercises (i.e., assumes behavioral responsibility to manage the disease), then one can live a normal healthy life.

Because clients enrolled in a partial hospital treatment program are likely to be involved in more than one concurrent group experience, clarification of how skills training groups differ from other groups can be especially important. Many clients tend to assume that all group treatments are simply forums where feelings are discussed. Although it is important that the group therapists not be perceived as uninterested in clients' needs and feelings, the quantity of material to be covered in any given group session requires that therapists "keep up the pace." A mix of supportive therapy along with the structured behavioral procedures is always desirable, and seasoned therapists can usually establish the necessary balance in this regard.

Communication with Other Staff Members

Our therapists have found it most helpful to read clients' charts on a routine basis and to attend the unit's clinical care planning meetings. This enables them to know what is going on with clients on a day-to-day basis, as well as what shape the larger treatment plan is taking. Such information may provide therapists with case material and examples that can be used in groups. By attending these meetings, therapists can add their input into clients' treatment plans and better integrate this aspect of treatment into each client's overall plan.

It is also helpful if therapists make notes in the chart about clients' progress in groups at least twice weekly, as well as whenever something particularly noteworthy happens in a group session. Good communication among all persons involved in the treatment process fosters better client care, and skills training therapists have the same obligation in this regard as all other members of the treatment team.

OUTPATIENT AND AFTERCARE CONSIDERATIONS

Rationale for Outpatient Treatment

We have utilized the skills training programs of Chapters 3 and 4 in outpatient settings, and as aftercare following partial hospital, residential, or inpatient treatment. We do not recommend conducting CET in nonintensive outpatient settings, however, because any residual urges need to be dealt with before the client leaves.

The primary advantages associated with outpatient treatment are the considerable opportunities for interaction between the treatment program and the realities of each client's daily existence. As clients are confronted with the stresses of everyday living, particularly the inevitable drinking cues and tempting opportunities to drink, previously unsuspected triggers for drinking or coping inadequacies may be revealed that require skills training. The events of clients' daily lives can be examined in treatment sessions and used as the basis for skills training, problem-solving exercises, role plays, and homework assignments. Homework can be tailored to provide practice in using new coping skills in real-life situations between sessions, whether on the job, within the family, or in other interpersonal interactions. This greatly enhances generalization of new behaviors to various aspects of a client's natural environment. The opportunity to practice skills in real situations is a major advantage of outpatient over residential treatment.

Outpatient care also meets a basic need for ongoing support as clients struggle to deal with problems in their lives, and with cravings and temptations to drink. In the event of a relapse, outpatient treatment allows for early intervention in the relapse process.

Of course, some of the advantages of outpatient treatment are also limitations. Relapse is a substantial risk, because clients have considerable exposure in their natural environment to cues associated with drinking and to opportunities to drink. Greater exposure to life problems and stress in the natural environment may also trigger relapse. Finally, distractions or resistance to treatment can easily interfere with clients' attendance at outpatient sessions and homework compliance.

Structure of Sessions

The usual length of weekly outpatient sessions is 90 minutes. Although the topics covered in each session are intended to teach skills relevant to the problems and needs of clients' daily lives, it is extremely unlikely that the problems clients actually encounter during the period of their treatment will occur in the sequence in which our topics are presented. Rigid adherence to an agenda of topics may lead to the perception that the skills being taught are irrelevant to clients' current needs. To help clients cope with immediate problems, and to encourage them to view the group as relevant to their daily lives, a period of supportive therapy is offered at the beginning of each group meeting. As clients take turns discussing problems they are having, other group members offer suggestions for dealing with them. Therapists structure this opening discussion along cognitive-behavioral lines, using a problem-solving strategy, engaging in functional analysis, and, as much as possible, building on skills developed in earlier sessions.

There is frequently conflict between the desire of clients to get help with their immediate problems, and perhaps also to "show and tell" to some extent about their daily lives, and the desire of the therapists to get on with the day's agenda. Often, the first phase of a session lasts 30–45 minutes, which is longer than the therapists would like but shorter than the clients desire. Clients are reminded that this time-limited group cannot always explore problems to the point of complete resolution. Where problems are persistent or seem overwhelming, recommendations for additional treatment are made (e.g., family therapy, individual counseling).

Closed versus Open Groups

One decision that must be made prior to beginning an outpatient therapy group is whether or not the group will be closed to new members once it is started. Nonreplacement enables the development of consistent working relationships and cohesiveness among group members, which clearly facilitate achievement of the group's goals. A closed group also allows for a consistent sequence of session topics, with later sessions building on material covered earlier. However, a closed group means that, as time goes on, the number of group members who attend regularly will decline. Also, financial realities in many treatment settings require rolling admissions to groups. Because each unit in this program starts "from scratch" in developing the "Rationale" and "Skill Guidelines" components, the program can easily be run with rolling admissions (open groups). In that case, part of the initial period of supportive therapy in each session needs to be devoted to introducing new members and guiding their efforts to achieve sobriety.

Engagement in Outpatient Treatment

Engaging alcoholics in outpatient or partial hospital program treatment can be a frustrating experience, because clients are at risk for dropping out. This section describes several procedures aimed at increasing the rate of client engagement and reducing dropouts.

One strategy that we employ to minimize early attrition involves having clients meet with one of their therapists prior to joining the group. The goal of this meeting is to allow clients to begin to establish rapport with the therapist and to learn how the group may help them. Many of the procedures described by Orne and Wender (1968) as anticipatory socialization for psychotherapy can be utilized in this first meeting. The assumption is that clients who get to know their therapist, and who understand the process and "rules of the game," are more likely to remain and succeed in therapy.

We typically have a therapist begin this preliminary meeting by providing general information about the program, such as the day, time, and location of the meetings; the duration of treatment; the names of the therapists; and the number of clients in the group. The client's major current problems associated with drinking are briefly assessed, as well as situations that promote drinking.

The therapist provides a rationale for treatment, drawing a connection between the client's specific problems and the potential for these problems to trigger a return to drinking. Clients are told that they must learn how to cope more effectively with these problems if they are to stay sober. The forthcoming group meetings are designed to teach the necessary coping skills. At these meetings, clients learn and rehearse new coping skills and are asked to practice them outside the group, between sessions. In explaining the concept of coping skills training, the therapist uses concrete examples drawn from each client's stated problems. For example, if a client describes a conflicted marital relationship, the therapist may focus on the units in which communication and anger management skills are taught.

It is important to anticipate potential obstacles to successful treatment, especially factors that may lead to early attrition. Therefore, the therapist explores any instances in which the client previously dropped out of treatment and advises the client that he/she should discuss with the group any thoughts of quitting treatment. Such thoughts are not uncommon, and the client may find that other group members feel the same way. Open discussion can resolve problems in the group before anyone drops out. Progress in treatment is not steady—there are ups and downs. Most clients at times experience hopelessness, anger, frustration, and other negative feelings about the group. Clients should be advised to discuss such feelings, even if they fear that it might be embarrassing to the therapists.

Many clients quit treatment after their first drinking episode. Clients should be warned that, even with efforts to maintain abstinence, some of them may slip and begin drinking. They are told that they should not come to group meetings intoxicated, but they are strongly encouraged to continue to attend group after a drinking episode, so that they can receive help in regaining sobriety, coping with their reaction to the slip, and avoiding future lapses. There is a delicate balance between setting the stage for clients to return after a lapse and actually giving them permission to drink. Therapists should take care that clients understand this distinction.

Managing Clients on a Waiting List

When closed outpatient groups are conducted with cohort admissions, clients often must wait for weeks before a sufficient number of clients is recruited to begin a new group. This waiting period occurs when clients most need treatment. In our program, we have attempted to minimize the wait by holding the first group meeting before the group is completely filled. We then add new clients, as needed, in the second or third meetings. This arrangement is a compromise between a strict cohort admission policy and rolling admissions. Clients who, under this arrangement, must wait for their group to start are contacted weekly on the telephone by their group therapist for support and assistance with problem solving. They are also called on the telephone by a secretary the day before their first meeting, to confirm the appointment.

Group Ground Rules

At the first group meeting, clients are given a list of ground rules called a "contract" (see Form 2.1 at the end of the chapter), which is reviewed with them, and which they are asked to sign and keep. This document is intended to enhance compliance with the norms and goals of the group, and reference to it during the course of treatment is sometimes effective in modifying a group member's attitude or behavior.

What follows is a brief discussion of these ground rules and our experience in applying them.

Attendance

Group members are asked to commit themselves to attend at least the first four sessions, in order to provide them with an adequate basis for judging the group's content, process, therapists, and members before making a decision to drop out. If they wish to withdraw after that, they are encouraged to discuss their reasons with the group before finalizing their decision. In our experience, this provision is often not honored, despite its being discussed with group members at the time they are recruited, at the beginning of group, and during the first several sessions. Most dropouts occur within the first 5 weeks, without warning.

Promptness

Clients are asked to arrive promptly for each group session and to notify the leaders by phone if they will be absent or late for therapy. This request is generally honored by those who continue with the group.

Confidentiality

Participants are cautioned not to reveal the identity of group members or specifics of what is discussed. However, clients are granted permission to talk in general terms about their experiences in the group, and particularly about the personal impact of these experiences.

Alcohol and Drug Use

Treatment participants are asked to accept the goal of abstinence from alcohol and all nonprescribed psychoactive drugs, at least for the duration of the treatment. They are also asked to talk in the sessions about any drinking or drug use that occurs, and about any cravings or fears of relapse that they experience. It is explained that it is common for clients to have some ambivalent feelings about accepting abstinence as a goal, and they are encouraged to discuss these feelings, as well as any actual slips that might occur. Clients are allowed to attend sessions even after an episode of alcohol or drug use, as long as they make the commitment to work toward renewed abstinence. However, they are asked not to come to a session under the influence of alcohol or drugs, because they would not be able to concentrate on or recall the topics covered, they might be disruptive to other group members, and they might undermine others' motivation or commitment. CET should probably be terminated after any drinking, however, because, theoretically, exposure-based treatments might not be effective in the absence of response prevention.

Although breath testing for alcohol has become common in alcoholism treatment programs, there are different philosophies regarding the circumstances under which it should occur. We have conducted some treatment groups with testing at the beginning of every meeting, and others with testing only at the request of the therapists. There are reasons for and against both policies. If testing occurs routinely, then unnecessary accusations and guessing can be avoided. Furthermore, therapists can avoid the awkward situation of discovering well into a session that someone has been drinking. On the negative side, routine testing requires some additional time at the beginning of each session.

The advantage of testing at the discretion of the therapists is that more trust may be conveyed to clients from the outset. Furthermore, time is not wasted unnecessarily. On the other hand, "spot" testing places the therapists in somewhat of a detective role that can be disruptive to group process. Regardless of how testing is implemented, a policy should be clarified at the first treatment meeting, and it should be enforced throughout the entire series of meetings.

In our program, anyone found to be under the influence of alcohol or drugs is asked to leave the session. This is done in such a way that clients do not view it as a punishment; anyone asked to leave is encouraged to return to the next session sober, and to continue in the treatment. In groups, the remaining group members are urged to share their feelings about the incident that same session and the following week as well. Clients asked to leave are not allowed to drive themselves home. Their car keys are taken away, and they are asked to arrange safe transportation with a family member, a friend, or a group member.

When discussing episodes of drinking or drug use with the group, it is to be emphasized that they are a common occurrence, and clients are encouraged to provide personal examples. An atmosphere of openness about this topic is fostered. Group members are encouraged to conduct a functional analysis of their alcohol use and of urges to drink, identifying specific people, places, events, thoughts, emotions, and behaviors that preceded and followed their drinking or urges.

Clients are given specific guidelines for dealing with the immediate aftermath of a drinking episode, including removing themselves from the situation and getting help. They are advised to get rid of the alcohol, remove themselves from the setting in which the drinking occurred, and call someone for help (their AA sponsor, a friend, their spouse, or the treatment program). They are cautioned about feelings of guilt and self-blame that often accompany a slip (Marlatt & Gordon, 1985), and are warned not to allow such reactions to prompt further drinking or drug use.

Clients are urged to examine a slip with someone, not to sweep it under the rug. They are advised to analyze possible triggers, including the "who," "when," and "where" of the situation, and anticipatory thoughts. Reactions to the drinking episode should also be analyzed, including behavior, thoughts, and feelings, with special attention to feelings of guilt, depression, and self-blame. Clients are warned about catastrophizing thoughts, such as "Here I go again; I guess I'll never change." The value of reminder cards, which list the troubles that addictive behavior has caused and the benefits that sobriety has brought, is stressed. Discussion of drinking episodes is designed to help clients plan more effective coping responses, renew their commitment to abstinence, and view such incidents as learning opportunities (Marlatt & Gordon, 1985).

Compliance with the requirement that drinking episodes be discussed in the group has been mixed. Some clients drop out of the group as soon as the first slip occurs; others keep it a secret; and still others use the group to help them try to recover from it. Group leaders must remain vigilant to avoid reinforcement of inappropriate behaviors that might "enable" future drinking, and to avoid allowing a lapsed client to get extra attention so frequently in the group that the client is encouraged to drink again. Specific remedial action should be suggested by the group members and leaders, and conformity with these recommendations can be made a contingency for continued participation in the group.

Length of Program

There was concern when we first designed our original 12-session group program that there might be a high dropout rate in an outpatient program of this length. In fact, in one of our clinical trials (see Chapter 1) there was a 40–60% dropout rate, most of which occurred within the first six sessions.

Although a relatively long program does make clinical sense, given the considerable number of relevant topics to be covered, the need for adequate time for all clients to role-play new skills, the need to review previous material, and the pressure from clients to help them cope with ongoing problems in their daily lives, it should be noted that longer is not necessarily better. Indeed, we have found significant reductions in drinking lasting at least a year when only five sessions of CET and interpersonal skills training were added to a partial hospital program (Monti et al., 2001). In another study conducted in our clinic, we had similar findings when only eight sessions of either CET or interpersonal skills training were added to a partial hospital program (Rohsenow et al., 2001). Clearly, when the treatments outlined in this book are adjunctive to other treatment, relatively few sessions can be very effective.

Attrition

Client dropouts are a significant problem in outpatient treatment for alcoholism. When recruiting clients for the treatments, we emphasize the importance of their making a commitment to attend at least four sessions. When the treatment begins, the contract we give each client reiterates this expectation, urges clients to remain for at least four sessions, and requests that they discuss any thoughts of quitting with the individual therapist or the entire group before acting upon them. At the first meeting, clients are also given an attractive wall calendar with all scheduled session dates for the coming weeks circled in red (Ahles, Schlundt, Prue, & Rychtarik, 1983). Whenever clients miss a session, whether they call in or not, they are contacted by one of the therapists to determine whether there are any problems and to urge them to attend the next session. These efforts are continued until a client misses a certain number of sessions or clearly states that he/she wishes to quit the treatment. When a client returns to treatment after an absence, he/she is urged to make future attendance a priority and to make whatever arrangements are necessary to avoid further absences.

In group treatment, absences have a clear negative impact on the remaining group members. They often worry that the missing member(s) might have had a slip, and this at times causes them to worry about their own vulnerability. There is also the problem, upon the return of absent members, of their having missed prior skills training elements. No special efforts are made to recapitulate prior sessions for clients who have missed them, so there are some group members who clearly lack certain skills. In our experience, group members rarely voice their displeasure about these problems to one another during the group.

Concurrent Treatment

Clients are encouraged to become actively involved in AA or Narcotics Anonymous (NA) and are frequently asked about meetings they are attending. AA is available for more frequent support, and a different kind of support, than can be provided by our skills training sessions, and will be available long after our time-limited sessions have terminated. Clients should be encouraged to view concurrent AA and treatment membership not as mutually exclusive, but as complementary (Vannicelli, 1992). Nevertheless, we sometimes see clients continuing with formal treatment but discontinuing AA involvement. For some of them, encouragement to go back to AA may have little effect until the completion of formal treatment draws near.

Some clients require professional treatment beyond what the aftercare group can provide. This has not been a source of conflict with clients' group involvement; often, these clients have less need to report on or receive support from the group for other problems they are having. Many of these issues are addressed further in Chapter 6.

Considering the Need for More Treatment

Approximately two or three sessions before the end of the group treatment, the therapists ask clients to assess their progress and remaining problems. Clients may wish to set new goals at this point. The clients' need or desire for further treatment, and various options for treatment, are considered. The therapists can provide appropriate referrals to another group, family counseling, or individual therapy. Continued involvement in AA and other self-help groups is also encouraged.

Planning for Emergencies

Major life events and life changes can be very disruptive and lead to drinking or drug use relapse. We devote one session late in intrapersonal skills treatment to helping clients plan ways of coping with crisis situations, such as social separations (e.g., divorce, death, child leaving home, close friend moving away), health problems, work-related changes, and financial difficulties. Life events do not necessarily have to be negative to trigger a relapse. Positive changes can also pose a risk, such as promotion, graduation, and moving. Therapists ask clients to describe life changes that they can anticipate and to consider the impact of these events.

Major life events can be considered high-risk situations that require effective coping skills. Therapists ask clients to prepare a general emergency plan for coping with a variety of possible stressful situations that may arise. Some of the skills taught in previous sessions may apply, such as problem solving, feeling talk, relaxation, and cognitive skills for controlling urges to drink; other strategies may include calling people for support, taking Antabuse™, and attending AA or other self-help meetings.

Coping with Persistent Problems

In spite of the fact that clients may have completed several months of treatment, they will certainly continue to face significant problems in daily living. We devote one session at the end of treatment to helping clients review remaining problems in their lives and develop strategies for coping with these problems.

First, common life problems are reviewed, including conflict or poor communication with family or close friends; social pressure to drink; and negative feelings such as anger, frustration, anxiety, depression, loneliness, and boredom.

Clients are then asked to describe problems that they had at the beginning of treatment, and the success they have experienced in resolving these problems. They are asked to describe the skills they have used to overcome or cope with these problems. Therapists press for specifics to enhance the opportunity for group members to learn from one another's experiences, particularly from the ways in which skills learned in the group have been applied to specific personal problems.

After recounting his/her experiences, each client is asked to describe the most troubling or persistent problem that remains for him/her. With help from the group, clients are encouraged to develop strategies to resolve their "worst" problems, drawing on skills taught in previous sessions. For example, a client may explain that although he has become increasingly assertive with his wife and is now able to express to her that he needs to have some time to pursue a hobby, he and his wife nevertheless are still having difficulty finding mutually enjoyable activities when they spend time together. Here, the therapists may suggest making use of the problem-solving technique as a couple, to come up with mutually acceptable activities.

Clients need to be reassured that they have the skills to solve life's problems without having to rely on the group or the therapists for support. Clients' self-efficacy can be enhanced by reinforcing problem solving that takes place between sessions.

During the last few group sessions, therapists should begin to "fade out" of their therapeutic roles. They should encourage clients to take responsibility for solving problems on their own. Thus, clients gain confidence in their own ability, which facilitates termination and enhances the likelihood of generalization and maintenance of the skills acquired during treatment.

INDIVIDUAL TREATMENT CONSIDERATIONS

CET was originally designed as individual treatment and was later adapted to a group format. However, the individual approach is easier to manage and allows greater ability to tailor the urge-specific coping skills.

On the other hand, the inter- and intrapersonal skills programs were initially designed for use with groups, but they can be applied to individual treatment situations with a few modifications. In fact, some of the units were adapted for groups from their initial development for one-on-one treatment. When a therapist is working individually with a client, a few elements of the program that were designed or adapted for groups will have to be modified. In the following discussion of these modifications, reference is made to the materials in Chapters 2 and 3, except as otherwise noted.

The ground rules, contract (presented in Form 2.1 at the end of the chapter), and goals are still relevant and important, but they will have to be modified somewhat to accommodate each circumstance. The therapist can tailor the program to the needs of the client by placing greater emphasis on certain skills training elements; omitting some modules altogether; and adapting the examples, role playing, and practice exercises to the particulars of the client's situation.

The "Modeling" procedures that are suggested in many sessions will each have to be examined. In some instances, the therapist can demonstrate the skills to be modeled, perhaps making use of an imaginary partner; in others, however, the modeling scene requires interaction between two actors and will have to be skipped. In those cases, the points that were to have been made in the modeling scene can usually be made when the therapist and client begin role playing.

Role playing ("Behavior Rehearsal Role Plays") is a crucial element of the sessions. Usually, when rehearsing a skill, the therapist will play the roles of other people in the client's life, and the client will play him/herself. On some occasions, however, especially when the client is extremely reluctant to engage in role playing, it may be helpful for the therapist to assume the role of the client initially, and for the client to play the part of the other person. In general, a client should not be any more resistant to role playing with the therapist than he/she would be with members of a group, although the client may find it a little more difficult to behave naturally when the expression of strong emotions is involved. This should be discussed prior to role playing to set the client at ease and reduce qualms about directing strong emotions toward the therapist.

The rule that therapists not spend large amounts of time lecturing to clients is especially true in one-on-one treatment. It is essential that the therapist solicit input and reactions from the client during the presentation of the Rationale and Skill Guidelines sections to elicit personal examples, engage his/her interest, and prevent him/her from tuning out.

Toward the end of the program, the therapist must be especially careful to shift responsibility increasingly to the client for analyzing problem situations, brainstorming, selecting appropriate coping skills, and so forth. In group settings, clients are forced to do this on their own to some extent, because not everyone can get all the individual attention he/she may desire; with individual treatment, the therapist should be careful not to allow the client to remain dependent on him/her. In CET, this involves asking the client to choose any skill or combination of skills to bring his/her urge down, rather than telling the client which skill to use. The process of fading out the therapist's initiative in spotting problems and suggesting solutions should begin well before the end of the program.

A final session should be used to review plans and possible responses to anticipated problem situations. Of course, the process of termination with the therapist is important and should be begun, as in group settings, several sessions prior to the end of the program.

FORM 2.1. Group Member's Contract

1. I understand that this group will meet for _____ weeks, and I have agreed to participate for that length of time. Although I do retain the right to withdraw, I agree to attend at least the first four sessions to give the group a chance. After that, if I want to leave the group, I will discuss my reasons with the group before making my final decision.

2. I agree to attend all group meetings and to be on time for them. If some urgent circumstance forces me to be late or absent, I will call [a telephone number is given here] in advance to notify the group leaders.

3. I agree that I will not reveal the names of fellow group members or details about their personal lives. Although it is all right to talk in general terms about my personal experience in the group, I will protect the privacy of others in the group.

4. I accept the goal of total abstinence from alcohol and all mood-altering drugs. I promise to talk in the group about any drinking or drug use that occurs, and about any cravings or fears of relapse. I agree to give a breath or urine sample if requested by the group leaders.

THREE

Coping Skills Training:
Part I. Interpersonal Skills

General Introduction   42
Structure of the Sessions   43
Introducing Clients to This Approach   44
Session: Nonverbal Communication   45
Session: Introduction to Assertiveness   48
Session: Conversation Skills   50
Session: Giving and Receiving Positive Feedback   53
Session: Listening Skills   55
Session: Giving Constructive Criticism   57
Session: Receiving Criticism about Drinking   61
Session: Drink Refusal Skills   65
Session: Resolving Relationship Problems   66
Session: Developing Social Support Networks   70
Therapist Tip Sheets and Reminder Sheets   73

GENERAL INTRODUCTION

This chapter and Chapters 4 and 5 provide session-by-session instructions for therapists who wish to apply a coping skills training approach to the treatment of alcohol dependence. The goals and the methods for each element of the revised training program are described in the detailed instructions provided to therapists in this chapter. Special considerations for clients with dual diagnosis are covered in Chapter 6, and structural and process considerations, in Chapter 2.

The skills training modules presented in this chapter follow a cognitive-behavioral approach to interpersonal, or communication, skills training. (In this chapter, the terms "communication skills" and "interpersonal skills" are used interchangeably in parallel with the research literature on this approach.) Communication skills are important for the rehabilitation of alcoholics for at least two reasons: (1) They can enhance coping with high-risk situations that commonly precipitate relapse, including both interpersonal risks for relapse and intrapersonal emotions such as anger or depression; and (2) they provide a means of obtaining social support that is critical to the maintenance of sobriety. Clients who began heavy drinking during early adolescence may never have adequately developed or strengthened these skills; these alcoholics will need considerable practice and feedback. Clients whose abusive drinking began after their adolescent years may never have applied these skills appropriately, or previously adequate skills may have fallen into disuse as clients became increasingly isolated with increases in drinking, or these skills may have become distorted as their social interactions became increasingly defensive and argumentative as a result of increases in drinking. For some, therefore, this skills training contains much that is new; for many others, it provides needed review and correction. In our clinical experience with the revised program, we have found that virtually all clients have found it useful.

The treatment manual that follows has been implemented by psychologists, physicians, nurses, psychology interns, and/or alcoholism counselors, alone or as cotherapists. The treatment has been delivered in both individual and group formats, with groups ideally ranging in size from 8 to 15 clients, but actually ranging from 2 to 30 clients or more. Although group treatment has proven very useful for the addictive disorders, the group format must be balanced with appropriate attention to the individual needs of each client. Effective treatment can only be provided by balancing the delivery of content material with adequate attention to process issues.

The topics are presented in this chapter in order of increasing difficulty and complexity, which is preferred when all clients can start a group at the same time or when individual treatment is conducted. However, in these days of managed care, we usually omit the first two sessions and conduct the other sessions using rolling admissions with demonstrated efficacy.

The program elements are presented in this chapter and the next in the form of a handbook. Each program element is intended to be self-explanatory to practicing clinicians, with a rationale and clinical protocol for every session.

STRUCTURE OF THE SESSIONS

The "Rationale" section at the beginning of each session is designed for presentation to clients and discusses the benefits of the skills to be taught in that session, first in general terms, and then as specifically related to recovery from alcoholism and prevention of relapse. It is useful to pose questions during this presentation to solicit group members' experiences relevant to a topic, so as to engage their interest in learning the new skill.

Next, the client is presented with the "Skill Guidelines" section. These can be written on a board in advance of the session to aid learning. It is important that the guidelines be presented as such, and not as inflexible rules. The goal is to teach specific coping strategies while encouraging a flexible application of them, consistent with each individual's goals, and with situational parameters.

Following the "Skill Guidelines" section in many sessions is an optional section titled "Modeling." Under Modeling, we present standard vignettes that can be used to demonstrate the skill guidelines. These can be conducted most easily if cotherapists are used but can also be done solo. First, a scene is described, along with the goals of the protagonist. Therapists usually enact each scene twice—once, contrary to the skill guidelines, and once again, consistent with them. However, many clients find standard vignettes less relevant and seem to benefit more from proceeding immediately to role plays of personally relevant situations, so these vignettes were not used in our recent clinical trials.

The "Behavior Rehearsal Role Plays" sections consist of individually tailored role plays that allow clients to practice the relevant skills in the context of personal situations they have encountered. In group settings, at least two client dyads should engage in role plays each session. The other group members provide feedback and support. Such feedback and support should initially be modeled by the therapists. After the targeted client has received feedback, he/she should repeat the role play to practice the recommended improvements.

At the end of the chapter are "Therapist Tip Sheets"—session outlines the therapists should bring to the session—and "Reminder Sheets" with Practice Exercises to be distributed as handouts to clients. The Reminder Sheets provide clients with a written summary of the Skill Guidelines, which they are encouraged to review at home and refer to as needed. The Practice Exercises suggest structured experiences that offer opportunities to practice the new coping skills in real-life situations. However, in some cases, the exercises describe hypothetical situations, which remove the demands of *in vivo* interaction. These allow more time for appraisal of a situation and the formulation of responses. Clients are expected to bring their written responses to the following session, where the practice exercise is reviewed. A review period at the start of each session provides clients with an opportunity to appraise their own behavior change efforts and to receive constructive feedback from the therapist, and from other clients in group settings. An overview of the session structure is given in a Tip Sheet.

Woven throughout the text of the handbook is additional material that we have found helpful, either in conducting our groups or in the training of our therapists and students. We have inserted this material where we feel it will be most helpful to practicing clinicians. To keep this information distinct from the handbook per se, we have "boxed" these points throughout the text.

A word is necessary about the style in which these units are written. The modules are addressed to therapists using this program, providing direct suggestions as to how to present the material to the clients. The text is worded in a "therapist's voice" as if a therapist were speaking with clients. Thus, the pronoun "you," when used in the model presentations and instructions within the following clinical protocols, refers to the clients (i.e., what the therapist would say to clients); "we" refers both to clients and therapists. Interrogatives are questions that the therapists may pose to the clients to stimulate group discussion.

INTRODUCING CLIENTS TO THIS APPROACH

In individual treatment, clients can be provided an introduction to this type of treatment in the first session. However, in groups with rolling admissions, a brief rationale may be presented whenever a new member joins the group, either by a therapist or by an experienced group member. Whereas new group members are sometimes quiet for a session or two, they learn through observation and quickly catch on.

The goals of this treatment approach may be presented as follows:

"We *all* have some problems getting along with family, friends, and coworkers; meeting strangers; and handling our moods and feelings. Everyone has different strengths and weaknesses in coping skills. Because alcohol is often used to cope with problems, interpersonal difficulties and negative feelings are often triggers for drinking and relapse. These triggers include such things as feeling frustrated with someone, being offered a drink at a party, and feeling depressed, angry, sad, lonely, and so on.

"An important goal of this treatment is to teach some skills you can use to cope with your high-risk situations. We will focus on ways to handle various difficult interpersonal situations more comfortably and honestly. We will teach you some skills and have you practice these skills while role playing one of these high-risk situations. In this way, you will learn to cope with high-risk situations and to prevent problems that could lead to drinking."

A key point to communicate to new clients is that the content of the program is tailored to the individual needs of each client. It is essential that clients leave this session believing that there is something in this treatment for them. The message should be "You will learn how to cope better with *your* problems." If clients believe the treatment is merely going to be an academic exercise, it will be difficult to convince them otherwise.

SESSION: NONVERBAL COMMUNICATION

Most clients do not need a separate session on nonverbal behavior, but aspects of nonverbal behavior should be addressed by therapists, and in every session. An occasional client, however, will need a separate session on this topic.

Rationale

1. Nonverbal communication, sometimes called "body language," plays a large part in the messages we send to other people. In contrast to verbal communication, which consists of the actual *words* used in speaking with someone, nonverbal communication refers to the *way* in which those words are projected. For example, during a job interview, one person might look down at the floor or off in the distance, whereas a different person might look directly at the interviewer. What different messages would these two applicants convey?

2. The same words will be interpreted very differently by another person, depending on how those words are delivered. In this way, nonverbal behavior can help or get in the way of the message you want to give. For example, if you fidget, rock back and forth, and speak in a whisper when you ask someone to repay the money he/she owes you, it is less likely that your words will be taken very seriously. Sometimes people say one thing with their words and something very different with their actions; that is, their nonverbal behavior contradicts their words, and the overall message ends up being very ambiguous. For ex-

ample, if you yell and frown while claiming that you are not angry, what effect will you have on your listener?

3. People are often unaware of the messages their nonverbal behavior sends. Some nonverbal behavior has become automatic or a habit.

4. Developing effective nonverbal behavior greatly increases the chances that you will communicate what you intend to communicate, and that people will respond positively to you.

Skill Guidelines

1. *Posture.* Developing a relaxed posture is important. Relaxed posture looks natural to others and feels natural to you. You should refrain from either slouching or sitting or standing too rigidly. Try to find a comfortable place for your hands (such as crossed in front, or in your pockets). Posture can convey shyness or insecurity. To avoid this, you should stand or sit directly facing the person(s) you are speaking with, or at no more than a slight angle. Being turned away from the person sends the message that you don't want to talk or are uncomfortable doing so.

2. *Personal space.* When conversing with someone, it is important to maintain a comfortable distance between the two of you—not too far away, and not too close. Each individual has a "personal space" of about 1 square foot encircling his/her body. [This may vary from culture to culture.] If this space becomes too small, the listener may begin to feel anxious.

3. *Eye contact.* It is important to initiate and receive eye contact while talking with others, by looking directly at a person's face. Not looking at a person while he/she is talking makes him/her feel that you aren't listening, aren't sincere, or aren't interested in the conversation. However, overusing eye contact can be as disruptive as underusing it.

> Be careful about cultural differences. In parts of American black culture, it is often the custom for speakers to look at listeners but for listeners to look away. Among Asian and Hispanic cultures, eye contact can also be interpreted as aggressive, rude, or sexually forward. Therefore, do not insist on eye contact if cultural differences contradict these recommendations.

4. *Head nods.* A head nod is a relatively easy and effective nonverbal behavior that lets your partner know that you are listening and following the conversation. By nodding your head, you can indicate agreement or understanding in a conversation.

5. *Facial expression.* Your facial expression should agree with what you are saying. A pleasant expression can help to loosen up a conversation by letting the other person know that you enjoy speaking with him/her. A habitual scowl or frown may be misinterpreted as disapproval or irritation. Being able to smile and laugh appropriately conveys the message that you are a pleasant person to be around and to engage in conversation.

6. *Nervous movements and hand gestures.* Nervous or distracting gestures that have become long-standing habits, such as playing with objects, tapping fingers, or shaking a leg,

should be recognized, so that efforts can be made to change them. These movements indicate to others that you are distracted or uncomfortable. Although hand gestures serve a good purpose when used effectively to emphasize the point of a verbal statement, too many hand gestures can distract from a conversation.

7. *Tone of voice.* A weak, hesitant voice; a cold, superior, demanding voice; or a flippant, sarcastic style can all affect how our words are interpreted. When making a request for change, a calm, caring tone of voice demonstrates respect and understanding for the other's point of view, whereas a cold, sarcastic tone of voice gives a very different message and is more likely to result in an argument.

8. *Timing.* This is an important aspect of nonverbal behavior. Eye contact, gestures, and head nods must "fit together" or the communication may be disrupted. For example, hand gestures may be appropriate in and of themselves but simply not fit with other aspects of the communication style.

Modeling

To demonstrate the effect that nonverbal communication can have on the impact of a verbal message, therapists should role-play the following scene using three different styles of nonverbal communication (and the *same* verbal content). The scenario is as follows:

> It is 9 P.M. It's been a long week, and Terry wants to get to sleep early tonight because he/she works an early shift and has to wake up before 5 A.M. tomorrow. However, it's impossible to fall asleep because the neighbors in the apartment upstairs are playing the TV very loudly. Terry decides to ask the neighbors to turn down the TV. He/she goes upstairs, knocks on the door, and says to them: "You may not realize it, but I can hear your TV downstairs in my apartment and it's pretty loud. I need to get to sleep so I can get up early tomorrow, and I'd appreciate your turning the volume down."

Using the exact same words, the therapists should repeat this scene three times with three different communication styles:

1. Hesitant speech, fidgeting, poor eye contact, apologetic tone of voice, slouched posture, and so on.
2. Loud, hostile, demanding tone of voice; scowling/glaring expression on face; hands on hips; and so on.
3. Relaxed but firm tone of voice; good posture; direct eye contact; and so on.

After each of the three scenes, the therapists should ask group members to discuss briefly how effective Terry's communication with the neighbors is likely to be.

Behavior Rehearsal Role Plays

Have group members generate personally relevant scenes in which they have had, or expect to have, difficulty communicating with someone. During today's session, practice and feedback will focus on the nonverbal aspects of the interaction rather than on the verbal content.

Introducing the Practice Exercise

Encourage clients to notice the nonverbal behaviors of people they interact with, and to practice using more effective nonverbal behaviors in their own interactions with others. Distribute the Reminder Sheet and Practice Exercise for this session.

SESSION: INTRODUCTION TO ASSERTIVENESS[1]

We have found that by having therapists be aware of the basic elements of assertiveness, these aspects can be addressed effectively within the context of role plays throughout the various sessions without requiring a separate session. With some individuals, however, it can be useful to have a separate session on assertiveness.

Rationale

1. "Assertiveness" requires that you recognize your right to decide what you will do in a situation, rather than giving in to what someone else expects or demands. It also means recognizing the rights of the people you deal with and respecting their rights.

2. "Rights" refer to the following:
   a. You have the right to inform others of your opinions.
   b. You have the right to inform others of your feelings, as long as it is done in a way that is not intended to hurt them.
   c. You have the right to request others to change their behavior that affects you.
   d. You have the right either to accept or to reject anything that others say to you, or request from you.

3. There are a number of different interpersonal styles: passive, aggressive, passive–aggressive, and assertive.
   a. *Passive* people tend to give up their rights if it appears there might be a conflict between what they want and what someone else wants. They usually fail to let others know what they are thinking or feeling. They habitually bottle up their feelings, even when the situation doesn't require it, and are consequently often left feeling anxious or angry. Sometimes they feel depressed by their ineffectiveness, or hurt because they wish others had drawn them out or figured out what they wanted. People have no way of knowing what the passive persons wants, and so they do whatever they wish, and the passive person seldom gets his/her needs met. In addition, others may come to resent the passive person for not communicating.
   b. *Aggressive* people act to protect their own rights, but in doing so, they run over others' rights. Although they may satisfy their short-term needs, the long-term effects of aggressiveness are often negative. Because they disregard others while they achieve their goals, they earn the ill will of other people, who may seek to "get even" later.

---

[1]This session has been adapted from Dean, Dubreuil, McCrady, Paul, and Swanson (1983). Used by permission of the authors.

c. *Passive–aggressive* people are indirect. They may hint at what they want, make sarcastic comments, or mumble something, without ever directly stating what is on their minds. Or they may act out what they want to say, such as by slamming doors, giving someone the "silent treatment," being late, or doing a sloppy job. Sometimes they get what they want without having to deal directly with others. However as often as not, people around them do not get the message and become confused or angry, so the passive–aggressive person ends up feeling frustrated or victimized.

d. The *assertive* person decides what he/she wants, plans an appropriate way to involve other people, and then acts on this plan. Usually, the most effective plan is to state one's feelings or opinions clearly, and directly request the changes that one would like from others, while avoiding threats, demands, or negative statements directed at others. However, a usually assertive person may decide in certain circumstances that a more passive response is the only safe one (e.g., with a totally insensitive boss), or that an aggressive response is necessary (e.g., in confronting a "pusher" who won't back off after several polite requests). However, what is unique about assertive people is that they adapt their behavior so that it *best fits the situation;* they do not always react in the same habitual manner to all situations.

Assertiveness is the most effective way to let others know what is going on with you, or what effect their behavior has on you. Being assertive often results in correcting a problem that is a source of stress and tension. Therefore, being assertive leads to your feeling more in control of your life and resolving uncomfortable feelings that otherwise might remain and build up. Your goals can't be met in *all* situations; it isn't possible to control how the other person will respond. Nevertheless, acting assertively increases the chances that your goals will be met, and you will feel better about your own role in the situation.

Skill Guidelines

1. *Think before you speak.* Decide what you are reacting to. What did the other person do? Try not to make assumptions about the other person's intentions. Don't assume that he/she must know what is on your mind.

2. Plan the most effective way to make your statement. *Be specific and direct* in what you say. Don't bring in extraneous issues. Don't put the other person down; blaming others only causes them to feel defensive, and they will be less likely to hear your message.

3. Pay attention to your use of *body language.* Make sure that your words, expression, and tone of voice communicate the same message. In order to get your point across, speak firmly and be aware of your appearance, your voice, your expression, and so on.

4. Give others your *full attention* when they reply to you; try to understand their point of view and seek clarification, when necessary. If you disagree with something, discuss it with the other person. Don't dominate or submit, but strive for a sense of equality.

5. Be willing to *compromise.* Others will work with you if you let them know that you are willing to work things out. No one has to leave the situation feeling as if he/she has lost everything. Try to find a way for both of you to "win."

6. If you feel that you're not being heard, you may need to *restate* your assertion. In some instances, persistence and consistency are necessary parts of assertiveness.

7. Changing a habitual way of responding requires conscious efforts and a willingness to endure the unnatural, awkward process of learning to respond in a new way. Someone who is habitually nonassertive will have to initially force him/herself to act more assertively. Otherwise, a nonassertive response will occur almost automatically. The first step in becoming assertive is to become aware of your habitual response and make a conscious effort to change.

Modeling

Demonstrate passive, passive–aggressive, aggressive, and assertive responses to the following situation: A person has borrowed a good friend's car for the day and has returned it without refilling the gas tank. The borrower returns the car keys, thanks the lender for the car, and enthusiastically starts telling the lender about his/her day. (A good way to start off the assertive response is for the therapist playing the lender to show sincere interest in how the borrower's day went and then to say something like "I'd like to talk with you about something; do you have a few minutes?") After each of the modeling scenes, ask the group what type of behavior was demonstrated and whether the "lender's" goals were met: first, to get the tank refilled; and second, to keep the friendship.

Behavior Rehearsal Role Play

Group members should generate practice scenes from among situations they have personally found difficult (e.g., refusing a request, expressing discomfort, asking a favor). [Note: Problems with criticism and anger are covered in other sessions.] Although the therapists have modeled several inappropriate responses to provide examples, clients should practice only assertive responses to strengthen that behavior.

Introducing the Practice Exercise

Ask clients to notice what their most common type of response is to social situations between now and the next session. Ask them to think about how they might respond more effectively. Distribute the Reminder Sheet and Practice Exercise for this skill.

SESSION: CONVERSATION SKILLS

Rationale

1. Friendships are an important cornerstone of everyone's life. In good times and bad times, it is important to be able to talk with and share with other people.

2. Conversation is an important first step in establishing both casual and more intimate relationships with people. It is a basic communication skill. There is always room for improvement in this skill.

3. Relationship between conversation skills and drinking or drugging and recovery:

a. Some people drink because they feel it helps them to talk to people at parties, gatherings, and the like. They may feel uncomfortable meeting new people or socializing without having a drink first. Thus, it is important to become skillful at conversing without first having a drink.

b. Some people avoid socializing or meeting people because of difficulty making conversations. This avoidance can often lead to loneliness, boredom, and feeling isolated, which are common drinking triggers (i.e., high-risk situations).

c. If most of your friends drink or drug, you may need to avoid them. You may feel lonely at first and miss socializing with drinking buddies. It is important to meet new people and to build new friendships, in order to reduce the temptation to return to the bar, club, or other drinking or drugging setting to socialize. The ability to engage comfortably in conversations is necessary for this purpose.

Skill Guidelines

1. *Listen and observe.* People give many clues that can help you decide what may be good topics for discussion. You may pick up clues from their conversations with others, or from things in which they seem interested. (How can you tell whether someone is interested or bored by certain things?) Approach someone to start a conversation when he/she is not deeply involved in some other activity, in a rush, or in the middle of an ongoing conversation. If he/she is in a group of people, wait until there is a lull in the conversation. Don't be hesitant and shy, but don't barge in.

2. *Small talk is OK.* Conversations should be fun, a way of sharing ideas or getting to know others in a comfortable way. Start small by picking a topic that the other person is able to respond to easily. Sports, the weather, asking who a person knows at a party, asking someone you meet on a bus or train where he or she is going—all of these are good, simple conversation openers. When you are engaging in small talk, let the other person know that you want to talk by making eye contact and saying something first, rather than just standing there and waiting for him/her to talk to you. Perhaps his/her coffee cup is empty at a party. Ask who he/she knows there, and suggest that you refill your cups together. Conversation does not always have to be "heavy" or "serious."

3. *Conversation is a two-way process.* You are not totally responsible for keeping up the conversation. Each person involved in a conversation should contribute about equally. Choose a topic that gives the other person a chance to respond easily and comfortably.

4. *It is OK to talk about yourself.* Some of us are trained to feel that talking about ourselves is not polite, and often we feel uncomfortable talking about ourselves for that reason. However, the only way to know whether we share ideas and likes with someone else is to tell them about our ideas, likes, and dislikes, and to ask about theirs.

5. *Use open-ended questions to prompt a response.* This easy-to-use technique is very effective in both starting and continuing a conversation. "Prompting a response" means giving the other person a natural opening in the conversation. An open-ended question encourages discussion, whereas a closed question can be answered by simply saying "yes" or "no." Examples include "What did you think of the movie?" versus "Did you like the movie?" or "How do you think the Sox will do this year?" versus "Do you think the Sox will win this year?" By asking open-ended questions, the conversation flows better.

6. *Watch the person's reaction to your conversation.* How is the other person responding? Are his/her responses to your questions getting shorter? Or is he/she throwing questions and comments back your way? Is the other person shifting his/her weight, looking at his/her watch, or looking past you? Or is he/she maintaining eye contact and leaning forward? If it looks as if the other person has had enough of the conversation, end it. Be careful not to overwhelm your listener. You do not have to say everything in the first conversation.

7. *End the conversation gracefully.* When your conversation is coming to an end, or one of you has to leave, you can end a conversation gracefully by saying something pleasant about how you enjoyed talking with (and/or meeting) the other person. You can mention that you have to leave now, or that you see he/she has to get going, and maybe you'll see him/her later. Basically, what is appropriate here is that you leave your listener with the feeling that you enjoyed sharing conversation with him/her, and that your feeling is sincere. This increases the likelihood that the other person will want to talk with you again.

> In our experience, many alcoholics feel that they are good conversationalists. However, in most instances, alcohol plays a role in alcoholics' confidence and perceptions of their skill. In the absence of alcohol, many of our clients have come to appreciate the relevance of the content of this session. Another important point is that situational demands can influence one's ability to use conversational skills. Attempt to explore a variety of situations with especially confident clients.

Modeling

Therapists role-play two strangers sharing a seat on the bus. These two people frequently ride the same bus in the morning on the way work, but they have never talked together before. Within this scenario, therapists should demonstrate the skills just described and show how use of them might lead to making a new acquaintance.

Behavior Rehearsal Role Plays

The first role play could involve group members interacting in the following scenario: Two people have just been introduced to each other at a party given by a mutual friend.

For subsequent role plays in this session, clients should use personally relevant scenes. Dimensions along which scenes might vary are (1) setting and (2) degree of familiarity. Is the other person a stranger, an acquaintance whom the client wishes to get to know better, or a family member with whom the client lives (and watches TV, etc.) but doesn't usually share much light conversation (e.g., about casual events of the day)?

Introducing the Practice Exercise

Therapists hand out the Practice Exercise sheet and explain as follows:

"By practicing these points on how to start, continue, and end a conversation, you'll find that those initial fears you had about walking up to someone and starting a conversation will lessen. You'll also find that it's easier and probably more fun for you. The effects of this lesson won't be immediate, but we all know that practice helps.

"Between now and our next session, you must, at the very least, start one conversation and record it on the Practice Exercise sheet. You are encouraged, however, to practice more than just once, whenever you have an opportunity."

SESSION: GIVING AND RECEIVING POSITIVE FEEDBACK

Rationale

1. The satisfaction we get from relationships with others depends partly on sharing *positive* things with them. Thus, it is important to be able to tell others positive things and to respond appropriately when they make positive comments to us. This applies to the relationships we have with all of the different people in our lives—with our spouses, children, parents, friends, neighbors, colleagues, coworkers, employees, employers, and so on. The types of positive things we tell others are varied. We might tell others that we like the color they chose for their new car, the way their new haircut looks, the helping hand they give when a task needs to get done, the way they lend an ear when we need someone to talk to, their enthusiasm when we take a Saturday afternoon off to do something fun together, and so forth.

2. Despite the importance of giving positive feedback for building and maintaining relationships, people often fail to do it. Perhaps they start to take others for granted, or they assume that the other person already "knows" how they feel, or they are uncomfortable giving positive feedback.

3. Some people who are very good at giving positive feedback nevertheless have difficulty receiving it. Likewise, some people who are good at accepting positive feedback have difficulty giving it. Alcoholism and depressed mood are often linked. If you feel bad about yourself because of past drinking, you may have a hard time receiving positive feedback. However, rejecting a sincere compliment can make the other person feel bad and may discourage him/her from saying positive things to you in the future. This may lead you to feel worse about yourself and make your relationships more negative. By learning to accept compliments graciously, you encourage others to point out good things about you and make them feel good about themselves as well.

4. How might the ability to give and receive positive feedback be related to your efforts to stop drinking?
   a. Relationship problems frequently accompany problem drinking. As the problems increase, the positive aspects of a relationship start to get overlooked. Making an effort to share positive comments with each other is one way to begin to change things for the better.
   b. Different people may be supporting your efforts to remain abstinent (e.g., friends, employer, family). By letting them know that you appreciate their support, you share a good feeling with them, and thereby also increase the likelihood that they'll continue to do things that are of help to you.

Skill Guidelines

1. *Whenever possible, state your positive feedback in terms of your own feelings, rather than in terms of absolutes or facts.* For example, saying "That's a nice shirt" sounds as if you're stating a fact about the shirt. In contrast, saying "I really like that shirt; I think it looks nice on you" conveys to the other person your own feelings. Even though both statements are positive, the latter will be more effective and more valuable to the person, because it is stated in terms of your feelings. Furthermore, a person's feelings aren't right or wrong, whereas a person *can* be incorrect about facts. It is easier for people to accept positive feedback that is stated as feelings rather than as facts. For example, if the other person dislikes the shirt, he/she can deny or debate the "fact" that it's a nice shirt. But if the compliment is stated as a sincere feeling, the "facts" of the matter become irrelevant; the recipient can appreciate and accept the expression of positive feelings as a valuable message, whether or not he/she feels similarly about the shirt. Of course, positive statements are valuable to others only if those statements reflect our *sincere* feelings.

2. *In giving positive feedback, try to pick out specific things that you like.* For example, if a coworker has been covering for you while you take a coffee break, it's more effective to say something like "You know I really appreciate it when you cover for me while I go on a break; you really are a nice person," than just to say "You really are a nice person to work with." Although the latter statement is nice to hear, it's probably hard for your coworker to know exactly what aspects of working together you like. Although general compliments are pleasant to give and receive, they are more effective if you also tell the person the specific things that you find particularly enjoyable or helpful. Specificity indicates to people that you have taken time to notice what they have done. It also helps identify to them the things they do that you find desirable, and makes it more likely that they will do them again.

3. *Accept positive feedback that is given to you; don't negate it or turn it down.* For example, if someone compliments you on a photograph you took, and you say something like "Oh, this dull thing? I think it's terrible. I was just using up the end of the roll of film and wasn't paying much attention to what I was doing," how is the person giving the compliment going to feel? Essentially, you are insulting him/her by implying that he/she has bad taste. You are implying that his/her opinion doesn't count for much, and the person may feel rejected.

4. Even if you disagree with the person's opinion, respond to it graciously and show *that you appreciate the positive feedback.* Accepting a compliment in this way isn't dishonest, because it doesn't imply that you share the positive feeling. It simply lets the other person know that you appreciate the compliment (e.g., "Well, thank you; that's very nice of you to say").

Modeling

Therapists may use the following role-play scene to contrast ineffective and effective ways of giving a positive feedback:

1. Guest *insincerely* compliments host(ess) on *entire* dinner that night. As a consequence, host(ess) enthusiastically offers to prepare the same meal for the guest again soon (much to the first person's dismay!).

2. Guest *sincerely* compliments host(ess) on the *specific* parts of the dinner that k enjoyed (e.g., the homemade soup and the dessert). As a consequence, host(e joys the compliment and offers to make those things again.

Therapists should solicit brief group discussion about the two different commu____ strategies.

Behavior Rehearsal Role Plays

Guide clients in generating and practicing personally relevant situations. Encourage group members to consider a variety of situations in which these new skills might be applicable to them (e.g., work, family, friends). Problem areas might include failing to give compliments, negating compliments, giving too many compliments at a time (thereby making others feel uncomfortable), and so on. One client should practice giving positive feedback and the other should practice appropriate responses for *receiving* positive feedback.

Introducing the Practice Exercise

Spend a few minutes helping group members to anticipate interpersonal situations that may occur between this and the next session that will provide opportunities to practice these skills (e.g., at social events, phone conversations with others, at work).

SESSION: LISTENING SKILLS

Rationale

1. *Listening attentively* when another person talks with us is very important if we are to get to know and feel close to him or her, and if we are to resolve differences.
   a. It lets the other person know that we are interested and understand what they have to say.
   b. It encourages the other person to talk about him/herself.
   c. It helps us to pick up on information that we would otherwise miss.
2. Relationship between these skills and drinking or recovery:
   a. Being intoxicated makes it nearly impossible to be a good listener, because it interferes with one's ability to concentrate and remember what the other person is saying. Although someone may have been a very good listener in the past, this skill may have become rusty through disuse. Thus, practice is important, whether people are learning or relearning this skill.
   b. Many drinkers report feelings of loneliness related to their alcohol use. Many people in recovery are lonely while trying to repair or build new relationships. At times, drinking is used to try to cope with the loneliness; learning other ways to cope with the loneliness will help to prevent relapse. Listening skills are one way to decrease loneliness, because they help you to build new friendships and to feel closer to your family.

Skill Guidelines/Components

Listening is more than just sitting quietly or passively while someone is speaking to you. It's an active skill, because it involves attending to and trying to understand what the other person is communicating, rather than just waiting for your own turn to talk. Practicing the following suggestions can improve your active listening skills:

1. *Use nonverbal behaviors.* Leaning slightly forward, maintaining eye contact, head nods, and sometimes a sympathetic touch or murmur all indicate to someone that you are interested and hearing what they say. Looking at your watch, yawning, or watching others enter a room not only distracts the speaker but also tells her/him that you're not very interested or tuned in to what she/he is saying. Nonverbal behavior is one of the first things that a person notices when monitoring how he/she is being received. Be aware that nonverbal behavior can vary depending on the person's cultural background. For example, in some cultures, maintaining steady eye contact may be considered rude.

2. *Think about the nonverbal behaviors of the speaker.* The speaker's tone of voice or facial expression may provide a lot of extra information beyond what she/he is saying. For example, you walk up to a friend and ask, "How are you today?" If the friend replies, "Fine," in an angry voice but does not smile or appears sad, then you know that your friend probably is not fine.

3. *Ask questions about feelings, paraphrase what the person says, and add comments.* This shows the person you are listening and understanding. An example of this is phrases such as "Wow, that must have been exciting," "Yes, it can be pretty lonely when you're all alone in the house."

4. *Share similar experiences or feelings with the speaker.* This is part of the pleasurable give and take of a conversation. However, it is best to wait for the other person to complete his/her train of thought before adding your own feelings or experiences.

5. *Timing is important.* The person who interrupts what someone else is saying because he/she is anxious to give his/her own version of the story isn't being an effective listener. Rather, listen for the appropriate time to talk, so that your conversation is a sharing of mutual feelings, as well as yet another way of telling the other person that you hear what they're saying.

Modeling

The therapists role-play two friends conversing about the skiing trip one of them recently took. The speaker, the one who went skiing, is enthusiastic about the trip and is attempting to share positive feelings about it (e.g., the relaxation of a weekend away from town, the freedom and exhilaration during a downhill run, the sense of accomplishment and pleasure after skiing down a difficult trail). However, the "listener" displays poor nonverbal skills, asks many annoying questions about the price of the lift tickets and lodging, forgets the name of the ski resort and has to ask again, complains about how it's always cold when he/she goes skiing, and starts talking about his/her own Florida vacation plans. In short, the listener fails to attend to the feelings expressed by the speaker, resulting in the speaker's waning enthusiasm and ultimate termination of the conversation.

The therapists ask group members to discuss briefly "what went wrong" in this scene and to suggest what could have been done better. They then repeat the scene, this time incorporating group members' suggestions and modeling more effective listening skills.

Behavior Rehearsal Role Plays

Each role play serves a dual purpose: One person practices talking, and the other person practices attentive listening. However, the focus of the role play should be on the listener. In some of these role plays, the listener can play him/herself rather than portraying someone in the speaker's life. Practice role plays can include telling a group member about an exciting meeting or lecture you went to recently. Get group members into pairs in which one person interviews their partner, then they switch roles.

SESSION: GIVING CONSTRUCTIVE CRITICISM

> Several sessions in this program focus on problems due to differences or conflict with other people, and the angry feelings that may accompany them. Two sessions in this chapter provide an opportunity to practice skills for giving and receiving critical feedback, a third session introduces the assertive skills necessary for effective communication, and a session in Chapter 4 addresses coping with anger. Because criticism is often viewed as a wholly negative or unpleasant event, an important goal of this session is to present criticism as a potentially *constructive* communication skill that can produce *positive* results for both parties involved. In some treatment sites, the word "feedback" is used instead of "criticism," to emphasize the helpful rather than the harmful intent of the information and style with which it should be presented.

Rationale

1. People sometimes do things that we find disagreeable or objectionable. It is important to be able to tell people about these negative things, and to request changes, without hurting their feelings unduly and producing needless fights and arguments.

2. Telling people negative things is often very difficult for many of us. Some people fail to give criticism because they feel that to do so is "not nice," and they wish to avoid hurting the other person's feelings, whereas others fail to give criticism because they feel that it's better to live with the unpleasant behavior than to risk losing their tempers or starting a fight. This reluctance to give criticism is usually the result of years of experience with *destructive criticism*—criticism intended to hurt. The skills we practice in this session are intended to help you give *constructive criticism*—to seek changes in someone's objectionable behavior without unnecessarily hurting their feelings or starting an argument.

3. There are several reasons for learning to give constructive criticism:

    a. By repeatedly not giving someone constructive criticism when it is called for, you are likely to end up feeling stressed and uncomfortable with the other person, then angry, frustrated, or resentful. These feelings will probably be reflected in how you act toward the person.

    b. Being able to give constructive criticism may not only result in positive changes in the annoying behavior but may also help you and the other person feel good about your ability to discuss potentially difficult topics with each other.

4. Relationship between this skill and problem drinking:

    a. The bucket principle: Many people don't deal with irritation, saying it's too small a thing to bother with, or it's not worth it to ask someone to change. [Draw a bucket on the board to fill with minor irritations that are shown with horizontal lines.] So they put the irritation in their bucket and it stays there. Then something else happens, and they put that in their bucket. These little things build up, until the bucket is full. What happens when the next irritation occurs? That's right, the bucket overflows. You may explode with anger or go out and get drunk or high. It is important to realize that when you do not deal with irritations, they do not go away. If you give critical feedback gently, when the problem is still small, you increase your chances of responding calmly and expressing your complaint in a way that the other person will understand.

    b. Many drinkers report that they cannot deliver criticism without having something to drink first. By practicing the delivery of constructive criticism while sober, these individuals will be less likely to drink.

    c. Other drinkers report that rather than give criticism, they deal with problems by becoming intoxicated or leaving to go to a bar. Anger, frustration, and resentment are common high-risk situations for relapse. Practice at giving constructive criticism makes it less likely that you will respond to objectionable behavior by drinking.

Skill Guidelines

    1. *Calm down first.* If you are feeling very angry or feel that you are on a short fuse, take a minute to slow down and become calm before speaking.

    2. *State the criticism in terms of your own feelings, not in terms of facts or absolutes.* Consider the following example: You have gone to a party with your spouse or a friend. However, when you arrive at the party, your partner leaves you alone, seems to be entirely absorbed in what is going on at the party, and is not paying any attention to you. If you say to him/her, "How can you just ignore me like that? That's the rudest thing anyone could ever do!", then you are stating the criticism in terms of facts or absolutes. In contrast, saying something like "When you ignore me, it makes me feel as though you don't want to be here with me," is a way of stating the criticism in terms of your own feelings. It's less likely to make the other person feel defensive and start a fight. A good way to remember how to state the criticism in terms of your own feelings is to use the following type of phrase: "When you do X, I feel Y." Notice how this is different from saying "X is a bad thing to do." By feelings, we mean some emotion such as angry, sad or tense. Saying "I feel that _____" is not a statement of feelings; it is a statement of opinion.

3. *Give the criticism in a clear and firm, but not angry, tone of voice.* If criticism is given during an emotional outburst, it is less likely to be heard and to be effective. Sarcasm or anger may effectively punish the other person, but that is not the goal of constructive criticism.

4. *Direct your criticism at the person's behavior, not at the entire person.* We can all accept that we may do various things that might be annoying to other people. However, it is more difficult to accept criticism if someone criticizes us personally and calls us names. Then, we are more likely to get defensive and to argue. Objectionable behavior does not make someone a bad person, so the criticism should not be a global attack, implying that everything about him/her is bad. For example, imagine that you come home from work and find that your spouse has left dirty dishes all over the kitchen. There is a family rule that dishes will be rinsed off and left in the sink after they have been used. You go over to your spouse and say, "You big slob. What kind of a lazy oaf are you? I think you must have been raised in a barn." What effect is this likely to have on your spouse and on the relationship? Because this criticism is directed at the person him/herself, it is likely to cause needless bad feelings and fights, and the spouse is very unlikely to change his/her behavior. The following way of giving the criticism focuses on the behavior and not on the person: "I don't like to come home from work and find dirty dishes all over the kitchen. We have agreed that dirty dishes will be rinsed off and put in the sink. I'd appreciate it if you'd remember to rinse them off and put them in the sink when you're done with them."

5. *Request a specific behavior change.* Sometimes we assume that other people know what they should do in order to please us. However, sometimes they don't know. What may seem completely obvious to us may not be at all obvious to others, and what seems to be stubbornness to us may simply be other persons' lack of knowledge about what we prefer that they do. So besides stating your feelings about a particular behavior, you also need to tell the person specifically what you would like to have happen. For example, saying "I'd like you to ask me my opinion more often" is much more informative and specific than simply saying "I feel bad when you show no respect for my point of view." "You don't care about me!" is much less constructive than "You didn't talk to me after work, and I wish you would."

6. *Stick to one point.* Many people try to address many different criticisms at once. In this way, none of the individual concerns gets resolved. "I'd like you to take out the trash each week. Furthermore, I wish you'd help with the vacuuming, do the dishes, get a better job, take me out more, talk with your son about his music," and so on. The other person will likely get mad or be overwhelmed and not deal with any of those issues. Deal with only one point at a time and stick with it. Try to focus on the future and resist discussing past issues. The point is to get the person to change the next time the situation comes up; it is not productive to spend time blaming.

7. *Be willing to work out a compromise with the person.* The goal isn't to "win" a battle but to reach a mutually satisfying resolution. For example, you may be annoyed at your sister because she frequently asks you to babysit for her and then returns home many hours after she said she would. Instead of insisting that she *always* limit her outings to short periods of time or *never* ask you to babysit at all, you might work out a compromise wherein you agree to babysit for longer intervals on a once-a-month basis, at a time convenient to you, and with plenty of advance notice.

8. *Start and finish the conversation on a positive note.* People are more willing to accept negative feedback and do something about it if they first have some positive interaction with the persons giving the feedback. For example, a supervisor criticizing an employee might phrase it as follows: "You know, you've been doing really excellent work lately, so I was surprised when you turned in that job yesterday with several mistakes in it. It's going to have to be redone, but I'm sure a good worker like yourself will be able to make the necessary corrections." Similarly, finishing the conversation with a positive comment makes it a more pleasant interaction for both parties and conveys the message that the disturbing behavior hasn't adversely affected the entire relationship. For example, one friend says to another, "Thanks for agreeing to share the driving sometimes. I'm glad we could talk together about this. One thing I like about our friendship is that we can talk about things that bother us." Make a sandwich by putting the criticism between two positives.

9. *Constructive criticism is designed to help, not to hurt.* Therefore, the wording should be specific and to the point but not intended to hurt. "You're a slob!" is not as effective as "I wish you wouldn't leave your socks lying around."

Modeling

Therapists role-play people who live together and both get ready to go to work at the same time in the morning. One of them often has to rush and is late to work, because the other uses the bathroom first and spends a long time showering, shaving, and so on. The one who is always rushed is annoyed at the other's behavior and decides to say something about it.

Scene 1: Demonstration of *destructive/aggressive* criticism: banging on bathroom door, yelling through door, name-calling, and the like.

After Scene 1, the therapists ask group members to describe what went wrong, to imagine the likely consequences of such an interaction, and to suggest specific, constructive alternative behaviors. The therapists then implement these suggestions in Scene 2 to contrast constructive criticism with the prior destructive criticism.

Scene 2: Demonstration of *constructive/assertive* criticism: better timing of the request (not during the morning rush), beginning and ending on a positive note, requesting specific behavior change, criticizing the behavior and not the person, and so forth.

Behavior Rehearsal Role Plays

Because receiving criticism is not covered until the next session, some group members may feel uncomfortable role-playing the recipient of the criticism in the present session. This may be handled in the following manner:

1. Therapists should acknowledge that this discomfort may arise and stress that the recipient is not expected to demonstrate a skilled response yet. Besides, this may depict a more typical example of what group members will encounter in the "real world," because most of their acquaintances will not have had similar communication skills training. In ad-

dition, any discomfort the role-play recipient experiences can be shared with the group and the protagonist, as valuable feedback after the role play.

2. Therapists may role-play the recipients of the criticism, if there is difficulty in having other group members play recipients.

Group members should be encouraged to generate a variety of relevant types of scenes (e.g., with family, coworkers, friends, waiter, car mechanic) in which they wish to give negative feedback.

Some alcoholics respond to problems with others either passively or aggressively. This may be due to their lability during drinking and/or the "black-or-white" nature of their behavior when sober (e.g., passive) versus drunk (e.g., "blowing up," aggressive). Because of these past extremes of behavior, we have noticed a tendency among some alcoholics to overcompensate to the other extreme when practicing these exercises, especially in the natural environment. They may be so eager to try out their newfound skills in assertiveness that they become aggressive, as an overreaction to passivity or vice versa. Therapists should gently help such clients find the middle path, without becoming too critical and thereby dampening clients' willingness to keep trying out the skills.

Introduce the Reminder Sheet and Practice Exercise for this session. Point out that the situation chosen for practice at home should be of moderate difficulty. Instruct group members to identify the person to whom they will give negative feedback, to set specific goals for the criticism, and to think about how they will deliver the criticism, *before* they approach the person.

SESSION: RECEIVING CRITICISM ABOUT DRINKING

Rationale

1. We often encounter critical statements in everyday life; one of the most difficult things to do in our interactions with people is to receive criticism gracefully.

2. Criticism, if delivered appropriately, provides us with a valuable chance to learn things about ourselves and how we affect other people. We all have room for improvement, and constructive feedback from others helps us to make positive changes in ourselves.

3. Relationship between these skills and problem drinking:

    a. Interpersonal conflicts, and the resulting anger or other negative feelings, are high-risk situations for relapse to drinking. Failure to respond effectively to criticism can lead to serious interpersonal conflicts, whereas an effective response can reduce conflicts and the probability of drinking.

    b. Problem drinking has probably disrupted your functioning in multiple ways (e.g., as a parent, spouse, worker). This has made you susceptible to a variety of criticisms about your behavior. This increased likelihood of receiving critical feedback makes it especially important that you be able to respond to criticism in a productive way.

4. Today, we focus on one kind of criticism—criticism about drinking or drugging. However, you can use these skills to handle all kinds of criticism effectively.

Types of Criticism

1. There are two basic types of criticism to which we may be exposed, and neither warrants an emotional or hostile reaction from us.
   a. *Constructive* (or assertive) criticism is directed at *behavior* and not at the person. In this case, the other person describes his/her feelings with regard to something you are doing and asks you to change in some way (e.g., "When you come home late, I start to worry that you are out drinking. Could you call me when you start running late, so that I know you're OK?").
   b. *Destructive* (or aggressive) criticism occurs when someone criticizes you as a *person*, rather than criticizing your behavior, or when the intention of the criticism is to hurt you. This type of criticism is often related to the other person's emotional state or is a provocation to fight, rather than an appropriate reaction to your behavior. Name-calling, or using words like "never" or "always," are examples of destructive approaches (e.g., "You're home late again, and I know that you were out drinking! You'll never change!").

Whether the criticism is constructive or destructive, it is not worth a fight. It is better to separate the *information* in the criticism from our *emotions* about the criticism, and not respond emotionally.

2. There are several ways people may focus criticism on drinking or drugging.
   a. Sometimes criticism about drinking takes the form of accusations or inquiries about "slips" (e.g., "You're home late. I know you you've been drinking again"). Even when you have made a sincere decision to stop drinking and are fully engaged in treatment, it may take time for others in your life to increase trust and to reduce their own excessive vigilance about recurrence of drinking episodes. You spent years losing people's trust, so you will have to earn back their trust over time. Sometimes the criticism is unfounded, and occasionally the criticism may be accurate. In either case, it is important to be able to respond to the criticism in a way that facilitates productive communication and does not start a fight. Similarly, even if the criticism is delivered in a destructive way, you need to be able to respond assertively and effectively.
   b. Sometimes the criticism about drinking will focus on historical events or on the negative consequences of past drinking. It may be either destructive or constructive (e.g., "You were a horrible person during all those years you were drinking. You wrecked our home and family" or "I'm happy about all the good changes you're making now, but sometimes I still feel sad and frustrated about all that we suffered in the past when you were drinking. If you would start to eat dinner with us again and listen to the children talk about their day at school, I think that would help me feel more hopeful and positive about us"). However the criticism is phrased, it is important to be able to respond to it effectively and to focus on

here-and-now solutions, without getting sidetracked into a nonproductive rehashing of past conflicts. Remember that you can't change the past, only the future.

c. During the initial period of sobriety, criticism about drinking may be occasioned by some behavior besides drinking that disturbs the other person. For example, your spouse may be upset about your isolating yourself in the den after work, or about your quick temper. However, instead of directly criticizing those behaviors that are disturbing, he/she may not mention them at all and may instead focus on past drinking or on present risk of drinking as the issue. This misdirected criticism may occur because drinking has been associated with those other behaviors in the past, or because it is easier and more automatic to criticize drinking than to focus on the other problems. However the criticism is phrased, it is important to be able to clarify the person's real concerns. This won't happen unless you can respond appropriately to the initial criticism and not get sidetracked into a discussion about alcohol when it is not relevant.

Skill Guidelines

The main goal in receiving destructive or constructive criticism is to prevent escalation into a fight. A second goal should be to try to understand the important information in the criticism and to help the other person to communicate the information more productively to you. Even some destructive criticism, although presented in an ineffective and potentially hurtful way, may contain useful information from which we can learn. Criticism gives us a chance to grow and improve.

1. *Don't get defensive, don't get into a debate, and don't counterattack with criticism of your own.* Doing so will only escalate the argument and decrease the chance of effective communication between the two of you.

2. *Sincerely question the other person in order to clarify the criticism, so that you're more clear about its content and purpose.* By asking for more information about critical statements, you encourage straightforward statements about your behavior. You try to get these restated in ways that are likely to improve the communication between yourself and the other person. For example, if a spouse criticizes you for going fishing, a nondefensive reply, which would help to clarify the criticism, would be something like "I don't understand what it is about my going fishing that makes you unhappy. Could you tell me what it is?", spoken in a calm tone of voice.

3. *Find something to agree with in the criticism, and restate it in a more direct fashion.* This is particularly important when someone is 100% correct in their criticism. Instead of responding with guilt or hostility, we can accept and admit those things about ourselves that are negative. For example, if you have not been drinking but your spouse says to you, "You're home late. I know you've been out drinking again," you might respond by saying "You're right, I am home later than usual today. I can see why you're worried, since when I used to drink, I'd often get home late." This approach takes away much of the negative impact of the criticism and allows the partner to be more objective in responding.

4. *Work out a compromise.* This consists of proposing some behavioral change in response to the criticism. For example, you run into an old drinking buddy named Charlie.

You make plans to go out with Charlie that evening. When you tell your spouse that you are going out with Charlie, he or she responds, "Why are you spending time with that guy? You know that he is still drinking!" Using compromise, you agree to see Charlie only at home with your spouse, or only at coffee shops or places where alcohol is not available.

Modeling

The therapists role-play a situation involving an employee who is being criticized by his/her supervisor. The supervisor knows of the employee's drinking history and treatment involvement. The employee has maintained sobriety for several weeks but has had a difficult afternoon at work today and has made some errors. He/she has had nothing to drink today. The supervisor points out the errors and expresses concern that perhaps the employee drank during lunch, and that the errors are due to the alcohol use. The therapists demonstrate an effective response to this feedback.

Behavior Rehearsal Role Plays

In generating role plays, prompt group members to consider various types of drinking-related criticism that they have received or can anticipate receiving. Responses to other types of criticism can also be role-played. Some dimensions along which the scenarios might vary include the following:

- The person delivering the criticism (e.g., employer, friend, spouse).
- Constructive versus destructive style of delivery or intent.
- Accurate versus unfounded criticism.
- A focus on inquiries about possible recent drinking versus past drinking episodes and their consequences.

Because many clients have received criticism about their drinking, the content of this session is usually quite familiar to most people in the group. Sometimes clients will have received the feedback while intoxicated, but at other times, they will not have been drinking. Because there is likely to be some emotional response to the content of this session, it is important for the therapists to be aware that some clients may be so angered by memories of inappropriate criticism that they may not hear the message of the session.

Clients' anger can be used as an opportunity for therapists to empathize with them about being falsely accused. At the same time, they can ask clients to discuss the reasons why others might be suspicious. This may help clients understand that the suspiciousness probably results from their own past behavior. Therapists can go on to gently confront clients about the fact that their erratic behavior likely resulted in lasting distrust on the part of others, and that it will take time and repeated efforts to earn back this trust.

Introduce the Reminder Sheet and Practice Exercise for this session.

SESSION: DRINK REFUSAL SKILLS

Rationale

1. Being offered a drink or being pressured to drink by others is a very common, high-risk situation for alcoholics who have decided to stop drinking. Have you received such offers or pressure? In what situations?

2. The social use of alcohol is very common in our culture, and it is encountered in a wide variety of situations and settings. Thus, even the person who totally avoids bars and old drinking buddies will still find him/herself in situations where others are drinking or making plans to go drinking. For example, family gatherings, sports events, office parties, restaurants, and dinner at a friend's home are only a few of the settings in which alcohol may be encountered. Weddings are particularly difficult because of toasting. A variety of different people might offer you a drink, such as relatives, dates, fellow workers, new acquaintances, old drinking buddies, and waiters and waitresses. The person may or may not know of your drinking history. An offer to drink may take the form of a single casual offer of a drink, or may involve repeated urgings and harassment. Different situations are difficult for different individuals.

3. Being able to turn down a drink requires more than a sincere decision to stop drinking. Specific assertiveness skills are required to act on that decision. Practicing drink refusal will help you to respond more quickly and effectively when real situations arise.

Skill Guidelines

What you need to do when offered a drink will vary, depending on who is offering the drink and how the offer is made. Sometimes a simple "No, thank you" is sufficient. At other times, additional strategies will be necessary. In some cases, telling the other person about your prior drinking problem will be useful in eliciting helpful support, but this is not always necessary. In many social situations, people will not even know whether you are drinking or not, and many people don't drink. You have a right not to drink. Stand up for this right.

1. Refuse the drink in a *clear, firm,* and *unhesitating voice.* Otherwise, you invite questioning about whether you mean what you say. Similarly, making *direct eye contact* with the other person increases the effectiveness of your message.

2. After saying "No," *change the subject* to avoid getting drawn into a long discussion or debate about drinking. For example, you might say, "No, thanks, I don't drink. You know, I'm glad I came to this party. I haven't seen a lot of these people in quite a while, including you. What have you been up to lately?"

3. *Suggest an alternative.*
   a. Suggest doing something else, such as going for a walk or a drive, if you want to get together to talk, instead of going out for a drink to talk; go out to the movies instead of going drinking on a Saturday night.
   b. Suggest something else to drink or eat, such as ginger ale, coffee, orange juice, dessert, or a sandwich.

4. *Request a behavior change.* If the person is repeatedly pressuring you, ask him/her not to offer you a drink anymore. For example, if the person says to you, "Oh, come on, just

have one drink for friendship," an effective response might be, "If you want to be my friend, then don't offer me a drink."

5. *Avoid using excuses* (e.g., "I'm on medication for a cold right now"), *and avoid vague answers* (e.g., "Not tonight" or "Maybe later"). Both of these answers imply that, at some later date, you will accept an offer to drink. However, excuses may be a last resort.

Modeling

The therapists role-play a situation in which the protagonist is offered a drink at a brother's birthday party. Someone hands him/her a drink and says, "Here, help us celebrate," and then ignores the protagonist's first refusal by saying, "Oh, come on, one drink won't hurt you." The therapists demonstrate an effective and assertive way to handle the situation.

Behavior Rehearsal Role Plays

Clients are generally quite good at generating appropriate scenes to practice in this session. Occasionally, someone can't think of any difficult situation. Encourage him/her to think ahead and to anticipate potential difficulties that could arise. As an alternative, describe a typically difficult situation for him/her to role-play. Some role-play scenes require using more than one role-play partner—for example, a group of people sitting around the table at a restaurant, offering multiple prompts to drink.

The role-play partners should insist and offer the drink at least three times. Initial role plays should be of only moderate difficulty, becoming more difficult as clients rehearse the skills. Include a variety of scenes involving coworkers, parties, restaurants, old friends, and new acquaintances.

> In drink refusal role plays, the client asked to play the role of the drink pusher often becomes overly enthusiastic in attempting to outsmart the client playing the role of the refuser. Although this may prove to be fun, and therapists should tolerate some bantering, it is important to ensure that more realistic and subtle situations are also presented.

Introduce the Reminder Sheet and Practice Exercise for this session.

SESSION: RESOLVING RELATIONSHIP PROBLEMS

> This session incorporates the skills taught in a number of other sessions, and in some ways therefore constitutes either a review or a preview of them. Included in this category are assertiveness skills, giving and receiving criticism, and giving feedback. Coordinate the application of these skills in response to problems that often arise within the context of close and intimate relationships.

Rationale

1. Improved communication can enhance interactions with other people. Sometimes it is more difficult to handle problems that come up in close relationships than in those that come up with strangers or acquaintances. Because close and intimate relationships can be areas of particular difficulty for people, this session provides further practice in using effective communication in these relationships, with a focus on marital or romantic/committed relationships.

2. Effective communication within close and intimate relationships is important for several reasons:

    a. It helps you and your partner to feel closer to each other.

    b. It promotes better understanding of each other's point of view and thus increases your ability to solve difficulties and conflicts.

    c. It decreases the likelihood that resentment and bad feelings will build up and affect other areas of your life as well. For example, bickering over finances or the in-laws may lead to more pervasive negative feelings and subsequent avoidance of sex and affection.

    d. Drinking and relapse are less likely to occur when you have an effective way to handle difficulties in a relationship.

> A discussion of communication in intimate relationships should address sexual issues, as well as other aspects of the relationship. However, people may be uncomfortable discussing sexual issues, especially in a mixed-gender group setting. Behavior rehearsal role plays on this topic may also be difficult, so therapists can present some hypothetical examples and didactic material on communication about sexual topics. The purpose of this is twofold: to sensitize group members to the critical role of communication within the sexual relationship, and to begin to desensitize clients to talking about this topic by addressing it in a comfortable and direct way.

Skill Guidelines

1. *Don't expect your partner to read your mind, and don't try to be a mind reader yourself;* that is, don't assume that he/she knows what you think, want, or feel without your telling him/her. Also, don't assume that you know what your partner is thinking or feeling. Because no one can read someone else's mind, clear communication about likes and dislikes is important. For example, your spouse comes home from work and slams the door. You might assume that he/she is angry with you. If your spouse says that he/she is not angry, don't assume that you are right. Think about the nonverbal behavior and ask your spouse about it (e.g., "Then why did you slam the door?").

Mind reading is especially likely to be expected with sexual topics. Partners are often reluctant to talk about things because they have learned to view sex as a taboo subject, or they feel they "should not have to ask" for what they like. However, failure to communicate directly about sex with your partner can limit the pleasure you both receive from your sexual relationship and can lead to unnecessary problems and anxieties. Sexual performance varies between individuals, and also from day to day, week to week, or mood to mood for the same individual (satisfaction can depend on position, amount, and type of sensual touching in addition to intercourse, type of atmosphere, etc.).

2. *Don't let things that bother you build up.* Frequent contact with a person increases the chance that some of his/her behaviors may bother you. If you say nothing about a repeated annoyance, irritation will build up with each repetition. It is important to give constructive criticism sooner rather than waiting until the annoying behaviors occur repeatedly.

Consider the following example of letting things build up: Suppose that, for a long time, your partner has not been doing what you think he/she should do to be helpful around the house. He/she usually comes home from work, says hello, and sits down to watch the news on TV. He/she expects dinner to be ready just as the news is over, and also that the house will be in reasonably good order by then. In the meantime, you have worked hard all day, too. You have had no time for relaxation. You have never complained about all the work you have had to do, or about your partner's expecting everything to go his/her way. On occasion, you have felt some resentment, but you have tried to overlook it, because you didn't want to start an argument. You have rationalized that it was "such a little thing, anyway." However, on one occasion, quite suddenly, you are feeling so tense and annoyed that you have a blowup over something very small. Your partner forgot to pick up the milk at the grocery store on the way home, as he/she had agreed to do, and you yell and say, "You never do anything around here; you're lazy." What are the possible consequences of such a blowup? How might speaking up earlier have prevented this?

3. *Express your positive feelings.* Many couples have difficulty expressing positive feelings within their relationship, particularly if the level of criticism has been increasing. Criticism then starts to occur in the absence of any expression of positive feelings, even when the criticizer loves the person he/she is criticizing. As good feelings get overlooked, and negative feelings become highlighted even more, this pattern can snowball. One reason that people become reluctant to express positive feelings is their feeling that to do so would contradict the criticisms they have made. For example, a partner may refrain from saying that a dinner is good if he/she has criticized his/her partner for serving it an hour later than expected. In reality, someone is more likely to listen to you if you have expressed your positive feelings as well.

A problem arises when we assume that positive verbalizations aren't important because "He/she knows how I feel, even if I don't say it." For example, suppose that after a hard day at work you feel tense, and you angrily criticize your spouse in a destructive way about his/her habit of smelling your breath for alcohol when you arrive home. Later in the evening, you realize that you were upset and didn't deliver the criticism in a constructive way, and may have hurt your spouse's feelings. You might say, "I was upset, but I love you and didn't mean to hurt your feelings by being so quick-tempered before" or "Even though I was upset earlier about your habit of smelling my breath, I know that it does show how much you care about me." Failing to express your genuine, positive feelings makes it more difficult for the two of you to work out problems.

A couple's sexual relationship is another important area in which failure to express genuine positive feelings can lead to needless upset. A common experience is when one partner is feeling very tired or stressed and is not in the mood for sex. If he/she only states his/her negative feelings and turns away, the other partner may end up feeling hurt and unwanted, and wondering whether something else is wrong. A more satisfying way of handling the situation would be for the less interested partner to share his/her positive feelings as well: "I really enjoy our touching and lovemaking, but right now I'm feeling pretty upset about some problems I had during the day, and I don't feel very sexy. I'd feel better if we could sit and relax together a while. That often helps me to unwind."

4. *Be an active listener.* By active listening, we mean use of nonverbal behaviors that show you are listening (e.g., leaning forward, making eye contact, nodding), thinking about what the other person is saying, asking questions, giving comments on what he/she said, and not interrupting with your own version of the story. This helps build closeness, affection, support, and understanding.

5. *When giving criticism, stick to the issue* (no kitchen sinking). Give specific feedback and deal with only one issue at a time. Don't throw in everything but the kitchen sink. Also, forget past issues and stay with the here and now. What either of you did last year or last week, or that morning, is not as important as what you are doing and feeling now. Remember that you can't change the past.

Modeling

Therapists can role-play one of the following scenarios to demonstrate the use of effective versus less effective responses.

> After a long day you arrive at home feeling tired. Your spouse greets you at the door and says, "I'm glad you are home. I told the Smiths that we would stop by their house later on for a game of cards." You reply. . . .

> You are at a party with your spouse (or significant other). Your spouse has been socializing with the other partygoers but has not spent much time talking with you at all. You feel bad that your spouse has not spoken to you much. You say to him/her. . . .

Behavior Rehearsal Role Plays

All role plays should deal with salient topics within clients' close relationships. A fair amount of time may be spent on scenes involving giving and receiving criticism, because these are often identified as important areas. Therapists should also prompt clients to generate scenes involving positive feedback, talking about feelings, and active listening, because deficits in these areas may otherwise be neglected. One strategy for generating role plays is to ask clients to think of interpersonal situations in which use of a particular skill (e.g., receiving criticism) would be beneficial to them. If clients have trouble thinking of situations, ask them to recall times in the recent past when they felt angry, anxious, or sad within a close relationship. This focus on feelings helps clients to recall relevant situations. Suggest particular communication skills that the individual might practice to cope with such feelings. Remember to evaluate the nonverbal as well as verbal aspects of each role-play rehearsal.

Introduce the Reminder Sheet and Practice Exercise for this session.

SESSION: DEVELOPING SOCIAL SUPPORT NETWORKS[2]

Rationale

1. Your social supports are those people in your life—family, friends, and acquaintances—who help you to cope with problems. Usually, such helping relationships are two-way streets, in that others also gain support and help from you.

2. Those who have a network of supportive people usually feel more confident about their ability to manage their lives and are better able to cope with problems. Research has shown that people facing a personal crisis (e.g., major surgery, chronic illness, job loss, death of a loved one) do much better if they have support from the people around them.

3. Relationship between social support and recovery:
   a. *There are many stresses associated with problem drinking*: emotional, interpersonal, financial, medical, and so on. Your chances of coping effectively are better if you have a good social support network. Staying sober, dealing with the problems that prior drinking has created, and managing the troublesome situations that used to trigger drinking are more difficult in the absence of support from others.
   b. *Often, people who stop drinking or drugging have friends who still drink or use.* When you decide to stop drinking, you may feel lonely at first and miss socializing with your drinking buddies. It is especially important to begin to meet new people and to build new friendships, so that you aren't tempted to return to the bar or the drug parties to socialize.
   c. *Some people feel that drinking or drugging helps them to socialize.* They may feel uncomfortable meeting new people or socializing without drinking. Some people may avoid socializing or meeting people because it is difficult for them. This avoidance is likely to lead to loneliness, boredom, and feeling isolated, which are common high-risk situations for relapse.

4. Many problem drinkers have found that their social support networks have deteriorated over the years because of social withdrawal, isolation, or interpersonal conflicts resulting from their alcohol use. Some people are reluctant to seek help, because it conflicts with a sense of independence or masculinity. However, a network of supportive relationships is the best way to support sobriety.

Skill Guidelines

After you have decided on a problem with which you would like some help, there are three basic steps to take:

1. *Consider what type(s) of support you would like.* This list may include the following:
   a. *Help with information, resources, emergency help or problem solving.* You might need information about local clubs and community activities, apartments for rent, available jobs, small loans, shelter, needed items, transportation, and so on. This

---

[2]This session is adapted from Depue (1982).

might come from someone who can expand your thinking about options and help you weigh the choices, or someone who has coped with a similar problem.

b. *Sober friendships*. It helps to have friends with similar experiences so you can compare your reactions to theirs and have someone you can count on for support with your sobriety. Sober friends may provide you with moral support and encouragement that includes recognition and positive feedback for what you do, as well as messages of understanding, encouragement, or hope. This support can be provided without actually working on problem solving. Often, this type of social support can help you to collect information and identify resources.

c. *Someone to share the load or help with tasks, as needed*. This may include family cooperation with household chores or help from a coworker in completing a job before a deadline.

2. *Consider who might be helpful to you.* This list may include the following:

   a. People who are already important in your life and usually supportive of you and your sobriety.

   b. People who might potentially play a more supportive role. These may be people you know or those you don't know well yet, including an acquaintance you haven't yet approached for help, an AA member, or a relative who knows too little about your attempts to stay sober.

   c. Be aware of people who are not helpful to your sobriety, even if they were helpful in the past. Some of them might become supportive, with some effort on your part. Most should be avoided.

3. *Consider how you can get the help you need.* Although dependable relationships take time and effort to develop, the following factors help to build a social support network:

   a. *Ask for what you need and be specific.* Let the person know how he/she can help you. Whether you are asking for help with a task, for advice, or for moral support, the more specific and direct your request, the more likely you will get the help you wish.

   b. *Be an active listener.* Whether you are giving support to someone else or thinking about a friend's advice about your own problems, it's important to pay attention and make sure you hear accurately. Active listening includes attentive nonverbal behavior, not interrupting, asking questions for clarification, paraphrasing what you heard to make sure you understood, and responding to the speaker's nonverbal message, as well as to his/her words.

   c. *Give feedback about the help you receive.* Your friends and family won't always give you the most constructive or satisfying help the first time you ask, even though they're trying. They need your guidance about what was or was not useful after they tried to help. Also, by thanking them for their support, you are more likely to get their help again. For example, you might say, "I really appreciate your helping me think through my choices objectively, even though you have strong ideas about what I should do" or "I know you're trying to make me feel better when you say 'It'll all work out,' but it would be more helpful if you'd help me come up with some ideas for what to do."

   d. *Lend your support to others.* Reliable support is a two-way street. A mutually supportive relationship is more reliable and satisfying than a situation in which one person always gives and the other always receives. Helping someone else out not only benefits the recipient, but it also strengthens your own coping skills.

4. *Add new sober supports.* For one reason or another, you may find that your current group of helpers does not provide the kind of help you need for the problem at hand. You may be the first in your group going through a major transition, such as commitment to sobriety or retirement. You need people who can give you an accurate picture of what to expect. You may simply wish for a new source of moral support, a person who will understand your situation. People usually enjoy sharing their experiences, and your first request may open the door for a new friendship. For example, "Hi, we've got a mutual friend. Joe Baker tells me you've just moved into a new sober house. I need a new place to live, and the house you're in sounds great. Could we get together to help me decide?"

Modeling

Therapists demonstrate ineffective and effective ways of asking someone to share the load:

Indirect request: "This clutter is driving me berserk."

Nonspecific request: "I could use your help more around the house."

Direct and specific request: "I'd feel much less pressured if we could work together to straighten out the house. Would you please sort through these papers while I do the laundry?"

Behavior Rehearsal Role Plays

Role plays may be done in the context of the Practice Exercise assignment. Ideas about role plays include asking someone in an aftercare group to give you a ride, asking someone in your meeting to be your sponsor, and figuring about a way to meet new people by asking a sober friend or acquaintance for ideas.

For people who do not have good supports, it is not easy to build them. A single session devoted to this topic only begins to set the stage for a process that may take months or years. It may be necessary to set the goal of building new networks within comprehensive, community-based supports, such as self-help groups and voluntary organizations.

Introducing the Practice Exercise

Leave plenty of time to work on this exercise during the group session. Ask clients to discuss and answer the questions in Exercise 1 of the Reminder Sheet: identifying a problem, potential supporters, and ways to get support. Also discuss the first two questions in Exercise 2: identifying someone who needs support and what help you could give. Clients should role-play ways to ask for and give support.

Therapist Tip Sheet: Nonverbal Communication

POINTS FOR RATIONALE

1. Body language and voice tone play a large role in communication.
2. Body language can help or get in the way of the message you want to send.
3. We're often unaware of automatic or habitual behavior styles.
4. Effective nonverbal behavior:
   • Helps you communicate what you intend to communicate.
   • Increases chances that people will respond positively to you.
5. Relationship to drinking or drugging:
   • Increases positive social and intimate interactions, leading to more support.
   • Decreases negative interactions that can trigger drinking.

POINTS FOR BLACKBOARD (IN CAPITALS)

SKILL GUIDELINES

1. POSTURE is important.
2. Respect PERSONAL SPACE.
3. Appropriate EYE CONTACT shows interest, sincerity.
4. HEAD NODS show agreement, understanding.
5. FACIAL EXPERSSION should match message.
6. NERVOUS MOVEMENTS, GESTURES show inattention, discomfort.
7. TONE OF VOICE should match message, show respect.
8. TIMING of nonverbal behavior must fit with other aspects.

Reminder Sheet: Nonverbal Communication

"Body language" can be very useful in helping you to get your point across.

- Posture is important.
- Respect personal space.
- Appropriate eye contact shows interest, sincerity.
- Head nods show agreement, understanding.
- Facial expression should match message.
- Nervous movements, gestures show inattention, discomfort.
- Tone of voice should match message, show respect.
- Timing of nonverbal behavior must fit with other aspects.

PRACTICE EXERCISE

Exercise 1

Between now and the next session, notice what you like about the nonverbal behavior of some of the people you see. List some of the positive things you observe. Briefly describe how those things may have had a positive effect on the communication process.

_____

_____

_____

_____

_____

Exercise 2

Start a conversation with someone. As you are talking, try to notice some of your nonverbal behaviors. Then, after the conversation is over, jot down those nonverbal behaviors that you thought you did well, and some that you'd like to improve.

Person you talked with: _____

I did these nonverbal behaviors pretty well: _____

_____

_____

_____

I could use some improvement on these nonverbal behaviors:_____

_____

_____

_____

Therapist Tip Sheet: Introduction to Assertiveness

POINTS FOR RATIONALE

1. Assertiveness requires recognizing your own rights and rights of others.
2. You have the right to:
   - Inform others of your opinions, feelings, in a way not intended to hurt.
   - Request others to change behaviors that affect you.
   - Accept or reject what others tell you or ask from you.
3. Types of interpersonal styles:
   a. *Passive:*
      - Give up their rights as a way to avoid conflict.
      - Fail to let others know what they think, feel.
      - Others don't know what they want so passive person's needs are unmet.
      - Result: Often feel anxious, angry, depressed, hurt.
      - Other people resent passive person for not communicating.
   b. *Aggressive:*
      - Run over others' rights while protecting their own.
      - Satisfy their own short-term needs.
      - Earn ill will of others, who then refuse to help them and might want to "get even."
      - Result: Long-term effects are negative.
   c. *Passive–aggressive:*
      - Indirect, using hints, sarcasm or mumbling instead of saying what they want.
      - Might act out: being late, sloppy, slamming doors, silent treatment.
      - Others get confused, angry, don't help them.
      - Result: Passive–aggressive person ends up frustrated, feeling victimized.
   d. *Assertive:*
      - Respect both their own rights and rights of others.
      - Clearly state thoughts, feelings, requests for changes from others
      - Avoid threats, demands, negative statements, intentions to hurt others.
      - In occasional situations, the most appropriate response is passive (e.g., insensitive boss) or aggressive (e.g., with a pusher).
      - Others feel respected, understand clearly the concern and the request.
      - Result: More likely to get needs met, reduce sources of stress, better social relationships, feel better about themselves.

POINTS FOR BLACKBOARD (IN CAPITALS)

SKILL GUIDELINES

1. THINK BEFORE YOU SPEAK. Question your assumptions about others' intentions.
2. BE SPECIFIC AND DIRECT in what you say. No other issues or put-downs.
3. Pay attention to your BODY Language
4. Give others' replies YOUR FULL ATTENTION. UNDERSTAND, CLARIFY replies.
5. Be willing to COMPROMISE in working out a solution.
6. RESTATE ASSERTIVE REQUEST if you're not being heard.
7. IT TAKES PRACTICE before this feels natural.

Reminder Sheet: Assertiveness

Remember the following points in practicing assertiveness:

- Think before you speak. Question your assumptions about other person's intentions.
- Be specific and direct in what you say. No side issues. No put-downs.
- Pay attention to your body language.
- Be sure you understand other person's point of view.
- Be willing to compromise.
- Restate your assertion if you feel that you're not being heard.
- It takes practice before this feels natural.

PRACTICE EXERCISE

This exercise is to help you become aware of your style of handling various social situations. The four common response styles are passive, aggressive, passive–aggressive, and assertive.

Pick three different social situations prior to the next session. Write brief descriptions of them and your response to them. Then, decide which of the four common response styles best describes your response.

Situation 1: _____

_____

Your response: _____

_____

_____

Circle response style: passive, aggressive, passive–aggressive, assertive

Situation 2: _____

_____

Your response: _____

_____

_____

Circle response style: passive, aggressive, passive–aggressive, assertive

Situation 3: _____

_____

Your response: _____

_____

_____

Circle response style: passive, aggressive, passive–aggressive, assertive

Therapist Tip Sheet: Conversation Skills

POINTS FOR RATIONALE

1. Friendships are important.
2. Conversation is the first step in casual and intimate relationships.
3. There is always room for improvement.
4. Relationship to drinking or drugging:
   - Some find it hard to converse without drinking first: you need to be able to converse comfortably.
   - Some avoid socializing because it's hard to have conversations: leads to loneliness.
   - If most of your friends drink/drug, you need to build new friendships.

POINTS FOR BLACKBOARD (IN CAPITALS)

SKILL GUIDELINES

1. LISTEN AND OBSERVE.
2. SMALL TALK is OK.
3. Conversation is a TWO-WAY PROCESS.
4. OK to TALK ABOUT YOURSELF.
5. Use OPEN-ENDED QUESTIONS to prompt a response.
6. WATCH OTHER PERSON'S REACTIONS and use the information.
7. END THE CONVERSATION GRACEFULLY.

Reminder Sheet: Conversation Skills

These pointers should make it easier for you to start a conversation.

- Listen and observe.
- Small talk is OK.
- Conversation is a two-way process.
- It's OK to talk about yourself.
- Use open-ended questions to prompt a response.
- Watch how the other person reacts and use the information.
- End the conversation gracefully.

PRACTICE EXERCISE

Start a conversation with someone you don't know very well, or with someone you'd like to practice having more comfortable conversations with.

Where did the conversation take place? _____

_____

_____

_____

What was the conversation about? _____

_____

_____

_____

What were the results of the conversation? _____

_____

_____

_____

Communication Checklist:

	Yes	No
1. Did you listen and observe prior to speaking?	___	___
2. Did you start with small talk?	___	___
3. Did you ask open-ended questions?	___	___
4. Did you share any of your own ideas, opinions, information?	___	___
5. Did you end gracefully?	___	___

Therapist Tip Sheet: Giving and Receiving Positive Feedback

POINTS FOR RATIONALE

1. Leads to satisfaction in relationships.
2. People often neglect to do this.
   - Take others for granted.
   - Assume others know how they feel.
   - Uncomfortable saying positive things.
3. Relationship to drinking or drugging:
   - Relationship troubles accompany alcohol troubles. Sharing positives helps change things for the better.
   - Different people may be supporting your efforts to stay sober. Show you appreciate their support rather than take it for granted.

POINTS FOR BLACKBOARD (IN CAPITALS)

SKILL GUIDELINES

1. State positive feedback in terms of YOUR OWN FEELINGS, not absolutes or facts.
2. BE SPECIFIC when giving positive feedback.
3. ACCEPT POSITIVE FEEDBACK; don't turn it down.
4. Respond graciously; SHOW APPRECIATION.

Reminder Sheet: Giving and Receiving Positive Feedback

Keep the following points regarding compliments in mind:

- State the compliment in terms of your own *feelings,* not in terms of absolutes or facts.
- Be *specific* when giving positive feedback.
- Accept positive feedback—don't turn it down.
- Respond graciously, show appreciation.

PRACTICE EXERCISE

Exercise 1

Approach someone and find something about that person to compliment. This can be done in the context of a conversation, or you can approach him/her specifically to provide a compliment. Afterwards, write the compliment in the space below:

_____

_____

_____

Communication Checklist:

	Yes	No
1. I stated the compliment in terms of my own feelings.	___	___
2. I made the compliment specific.	___	___

Exercise 2

Stay alert until our next session for any compliments you may receive. Try to respond according to the guidelines discussed in today's session. For one compliment that you receive, record the following:

Describe situation: _____

_____

_____

What was your response? _____

_____

_____

Communication Checklist:

	Yes	No
1. Did you accept the compliment?	___	___
2. Did you turn down or differ with the compliment given to you?	___	___
3. Did you show your appreciation?	___	___

Therapist Tip Sheet: Listening Skills

POINTS FOR RATIONALE

1. Listening attentively:
   - Helps us get to know someone, feel close, resolve differences.
   - Shows interest and understanding.
   - Encourages others to talk about self.
   - Helps us learn information.
2. Relationship to drinking or drugging:
   - Intoxication prevented good listening by impairing concentration, memory.
   - Listening skills became rusty through lack of use.
   - Many in recovery are lonely while trying to repair or build new relationships.
   - Loneliness can lead to drinking to avoid feelings.
   - Listening helps builds new friendships, feel closer to family.

POINTS FOR BLACKBOARD (IN CAPITALS)

SKILL GUILDELINES

1. USE NONVERBAL BEHAVIORS to show interest, listening.
2. Think about SPEAKER'S NONVERBAL BEHAVIORS for extra information.
3. ASK QUESTIONS, PARAPHRASE what was said, ADD COMMENTS to show listening, understanding.
4. SHARE YOUR SIMILAR EXPERIENCES OR FEELINGS after the other finishes.
5. TIMING IS IMPORTANT. Wait for appropriate time, rather than interrupting.

Reminder Sheet: Listening Skills

When listening to other people:

- Use "body language" to show that you are listening to the other person (leaning forward, eye contact, head nods, etc.).
- Think about the speaker's tone of voice, facial expression, and body language, to help you "tune in to" his/her feelings.
- Ask questions about feelings, rephrase what was said, and add comments.
- Share similar experiences or feelings that you have had.
- Listen for an appropriate time to talk. Wait until they finish instead of interrupting.

PRACTICE EXERCISE

Practice listening to others. Describe the situations below.

Exercise 1: Practice Listening to Feelings

During an interaction you have with someone, notice a feeling that he/she is expressing both verbally and with body language.

1. What feeling did he/she express verbally? _____

_____

_____

_____

2. What body language behaviors did you notice? _____

_____

_____

_____

3. What feeling was he/she expressing through body language? _____

_____

_____

_____

4. How did you show you were listening? _____

_____

_____

_____

(continued)

Exercise 2: Practice Listening to Conversation

Ask someone about an enjoyable recreational event or meeting he/she went to recently. Practice the listening skills.

1. What ways did you show interest by asking questions or paraphrasing what he/she said? _____

_____

_____

_____

2. What ways did you share similar experiences or feeling? _____

_____

_____

_____

3. What body language did you use to show you were listening? _____

_____

_____

_____

Therapist Tip Sheet: Giving Constructive Criticism

POINTS FOR RATIONALE

1. We need to say what bothers us and request changes.
2. Often difficult because of our experience with destructive criticism.
   - Destructive criticism: Intended to hurt.
   - Constructive criticism: Seek behavior change without needless hurt, arguments.
3. Reasons to learn to give constructive criticism:
   - Not doing so leads to more stress, frustration, anger, resentment. We then act angry/resentful toward the other person.
   - Constructive criticism can result in changes in the annoying behavior, better communication, both people feel better about ability to discuss problems.
4. Relationship to drinking or drugging:
   - Bucket principle: Filling your "bucket" with irritations until bucket overflows vs. handling them before they build up.
   - Many drinkers drink before giving criticism.
   - Many drinkers drink to avoid dealing with problems.
   - Anger, frustration, resentment are common relapse triggers.
   - Constructive criticism makes it less likely you will drink in response to behavior you find objectionable.

POINTS FOR BLACKBOARD (IN CAPITALS)

SKILL GUIDELINES

1. CALM DOWN FIRST.
2. STATE criticism in terms of OWN FEELINGS, NOT as FACTS OR ABSOLUTES. "When you do _____, I feel _____."
3. Use CLEAR, FIRM, NOT ANGRY TONE OF VOICE.
4. CRITICIZE THE BEHAVIOR, NOT THE PERSON.
5. REQUEST A SPECIFIC BEHAVIOR CHANGE.
6. STICK TO ONE POINT. Don't add any other issues or get sidetracked.
7. BE WILLING TO work out a COMPROMISE.
8. START AND FINISH ON POSITIVE NOTE. Sandwich the criticism between positives.
9. The criticism should be NOT INTENDED TO HURT. No insults or hurtful language.

Reminder Sheet: Giving Constructive Criticism

Here are some suggestions for giving constructive, assertive criticism:

- Calm down first.
- State the criticism in terms of your own feelings, not in terms of absolute facts. "When you do _____, I feel _____."
- Use a clear, firm, not angry tone of voice.
- Criticize the behavior, not the person.
- Request a *specific* behavior change.
- Stick to one point.
- Be willing to work out a compromise.
- Start and finish on a positive note.
- Remember that the criticism is not intended to hurt.

PRACTICE EXERCISE

Approach a person who you have been meaning to tell something negative to. Provide that person with some constructive criticism. Try to follow the guidelines outlined in the session.
Before leaving today's group session:

Identify the problem: _____

_____

_____

_____

Your goals: _____

_____

_____

_____

After speaking to the person, describe what happened:

What did you say to him/her? _____

_____

_____

_____

How did he/she respond? _____

_____

_____

_____

Therapist Tip Sheet: Receiving Criticism about Drinking

POINTS FOR RATIONALE

1. It is difficult to receive criticism gracefully.
2. Valuable feedback: can learn about ourselves and how we affect others, use it to improve and grow.
3. Relationship to drinking or drugging:
   - Conflict with people often triggers relapse.
   - Responding well to criticism can reduce conflicts and probability of relapse.
   - Problem drinking leaves you open to much criticism, so it is important to handle it well.
4. Use today's skills to handle all kinds of criticism.

POINTS FOR BLACKBOARD (IN CAPITALS)

TYPES OF CRITICISM

1. CONSTRUCTIVE (directed at behavior) VS. DESTRUCTIVE CRITICISM (intended to hurt, extreme wording, provoking).
2. SEPARATE INFORMATION FROM EMOTIONS.
3. Criticism about drinking can be ACCURATE OR INACCURATE: IT TAKES TIME TO EARN TRUST BACK.
4. Criticism can focus on PAST DRINKING VS. PRESENT BEHAVIOR.
5. CONCERN ABOUT SOME OTHER BEHAVIOR CAN LEAD TO ACCUSATION OF DRINKING.

SKILL GUIDELINES

1. DON'T GET DEFENSIVE, DEBATE, or COUNTERATTACK.
2. CLARIFY CRITICISM WITH SINCERE QUESTIONS until clear about content, purpose.
3. AGREE WITH SOMETHING, RESTATE IT IN MORE DIRECT WAY.
4. WORK OUT A COMPROMISE. Propose a change in your own behavior.

Reminder Sheet: Receiving Criticism about Drinking

When you receive criticism about drinking, remember the following:

- Don't get defensive, don't debate, don't counterattack.
- Ask sincere questions for clarification until you are clear about what is meant.
- Find something to agree with in the criticism.
- Work out a compromise:
  Agree to keep the criticizer better informed about your feelings and moods, your activities, and any slips you may have.

PRACTICE EXERCISE

Imagine the following situation: You come home from work after a long hard day. You've been sober for about 3 months and have had nothing to drink today. However, your eyes are red, and you're feeling somewhat "down" and irritable. Your spouse (or someone you live with) approaches you, smells your breath, and says, "You've been drinking again, haven't you?"

In the space below, write an assertive response: _____

_____

_____

_____

_____

Therapist Tip Sheet: Drink Refusal Skills

POINTS FOR RATIONALE

1. Drink offers are a common high-risk situation.
2. Alcohol use is common, hard to avoid. You must learn how to handle offers to drink.
3. You need more than willpower: you need specific skills, practice, to be quick and effective.

POINTS FOR BLACKBOARD (IN CAPITALS)

SKILL GUIDELINES

1. Give refusal in a CLEAR, UNHESITATING, FIRM VOICE; DIRECT EYE CONTACT.
2. After saying "no," CHANGE THE SUBJECT.
3. SUGGEST ALTERNATIVE activity or beverage.
4. ASK THEM TO STOP OFFERING, if they persist.
5. AVOID EXCUSES or VAGUE ANSWERS except as last resort.

Reminder Sheet: Drink Refusal Skills

When you are urged to drink, keep the following in mind:

- Say "no" first in a clear, firm, and unhesitating voice.
- Make direct eye contact.
- Change the subject.
- Suggest an alternative:
    Something else to do.
    Something else to eat or drink.
- Ask the person to stop offering you a drink and not to do so again.
- Avoid using excuses or vague answers.
- Remember: It's your right not to drink!

PRACTICE EXERCISE

Listed below are some people who might offer you a drink in the future. Give some thought to how you will respond to them, and write your responses under each item.

Someone close to you who knows about your drinking problem: _____

_____

_____

Coworker: _____

_____

_____

Boss: _____

_____

_____

New acquaintance: _____

_____

_____

Waitress/waiter with others present: _____

_____

_____

Relative at a family gathering: _____

_____

_____

Therapist Tip Sheet: Resolving Relationship Problems

POINTS FOR RATIONALE

1. Close and intimate relationships can be especially difficult to handle effectively.
2. Important because:
   - Helps you and partner feel closer.
   - Increases understanding, ability to solve conflicts and problems.
   - Bad feelings, resentment less likely to build up.
3. Relationship to drinking or drugging:
   - Effectively handling difficulties makes relationships better.
   - Less likely to relapse in supportive, rewarding relationship.

POINTS FOR BLACKBOARD (IN CAPITALS)

SKILL GUIDELINES

1. NO MIND READING. Don't assume either knows what the other thinks.
2. DON'T LET IRRITATIONS BUILD UP. Give constructive feedback early.
3. EXPRESS POSITIVE FEELINGS about other person.
4. BE AN ACTIVE LISTENER.
5. STICK TO THE POINT, one issue at a time, here and now.

Reminder Sheet: Resolving Relationship Problems

The following points can be helpful when working out differences within a close relationship:

- No mind reading. Don't expect your partner to read your mind, and you can't really read your partner's mind.
- Don't let things that bother you build up: Give constructive criticism at an early point.
    Calm down.
    State the criticism in terms of your own feelings.
    Criticize specific behavior, not the person.
    Request specific behavior change.
    Offer to compromise.
- Express your positive feelings about the other person.
    Compliment some specific behavior.
- Stick to the point. Talk about one issue at a time.
- Be an active listener.
    Pay attention to the other person's feelings.
    Ask questions.
    Add comments of your own.
    Share similar experiences.

PRACTICE EXERCISE

Think about a current situation that is bothering you with your spouse or another close person. Choose a situation that matters to you and is important to try to change, but one that is not extremely difficult. After you think of the situation, answer the following questions:

1. Describe the situation. (For example, "We sit at the dinner table and ignore each other.")

_____

_____

_____

2. Describe what you usually do or fail to do in the situation. (For example, "I usually read the paper and ignore my spouse while eating dinner.") _____

_____

_____

_____

3. What specifically would you like to try to do differently in this situation? (For example, "I'd like to ask my spouse about how his/her day was and to listen actively to what he/she has to say.")

_____

_____

_____

_____

4. Now, choose the right time and place, and try out your new behavior or skill in the problem situation. In the space below, describe the results of the interaction and how your partner responded.

_____

_____

_____

Therapist Tip Sheet: Developing Social Support Networks

POINTS FOR RATIONALE

1. People who help you cope with problems. Often a two-way street.
2. Leads to more confidence about ability to manage problems, less stress.
3. Many social networks deteriorated during drinking/drug use due to isolation, conflicts. Some people are reluctant to seek help due to independence, masculinity.
4. Relationship to drinking or drugging:
   - Helps in dealing with problems caused by prior drinking, handling drinking triggers.
   - Building new friendships helps to avoid temptation to see drinking friends.
   - Some people avoid socializing unless intoxicated, get lonely/bored, triggering relapse.

POINTS FOR BLACKBOARD (IN CAPITALS)

SKILL GUIDELINES

1. TYPE OF SUPPORT WANTED:
   - INFORMATION, RESOURCES, EMERGENCY HELP, PROBLEM SOLVING
   - SOBER FRIENDSHIPS
   - HELP WITH TASKS
2. WHO MIGHT BE HELPFUL?
   - WHO ARE CURRENT SUPPORTS?
   - WHO ARE POTENTIAL SUPPORTS?
   - WHO IS NOT HELPFUL?
3. HOW TO GET SUPPORT:
   - ASK for help, BE SPECIFIC.
   - BE AN ACTIVE LISTENER.
   - GIVE FEEDBACK ABOUT HELP GIVEN, THANK THEM.
   - GIVE SUPPORT TO OTHERS.
4. ADD NEW SOBER SUPPORTS

Reminder Sheet: Developing Social Support Networks

- WHAT types of support will be most helpful?
    - Help with information, resources, emergency help, or problem solving
    - Sober friendships
    - Someone to share the load
- WHO might be able to be helpful to you? This includes people who have been:
    - Usually supportive
    - Neutral, but might be supportive if asked
    - Not helpful, but they may become supportive with some effort
- HOW can you get the support or help you need?
    - Ask for what you need. Be specific and direct.
    - Be an active listener when giving or receiving support.
    - Give feedback about what was or wasn't helpful; thank the person for his/her support.
    - Lend your support to others; support is a two-way street.
- Add new sober supports.

PRACTICE EXERCISE

Exercise 1

Think of a current problem that you would like help with.

Describe the problem: _____

_____

_____

_____

Who might help you with this problem? _____

What might he/she do to lend you the support you'd like? _____

_____

_____

_____

How can you try to get this support from him/her? _____

_____

_____

_____

Now, choose the right time and situation, and try to get this person to support you. Describe what happened: _____

_____

_____

_____

(continued)

Exercise 2

Name a friend or family member who is currently having a problem and could use some more support from you. _____

Describe what you could do to lend him/her some support: _____

_____

_____

_____

Now, choose an appropriate time and setting, and give support to this person.

Describe what happened: _____

_____

_____

FOUR

Coping Skills Training:
Part II. Intrapersonal Skills

General Introduction   95
Session: Managing Urges to Drink   96
Session: Problem Solving   99
Session: Increasing Pleasant Activities   102
Session: Anger Management   104
Session: Managing Negative Thinking   108
Session: Seemingly Irrelevant Decisions   113
Session: Planning for Emergencies   115
Therapist Tip Sheets and Reminder Sheets   117

GENERAL INTRODUCTION

The coping skills strategies covered in this chapter can be divided into two general categories: skills for coping with specific, intrapersonal drinking triggers, and general lifestyle modification strategies. Skills for coping with specific intrapersonal triggers include managing urges to drink, anger, and other negative mood states, and planning for emergency situations. Lifestyle modification strategies include skills for identifying and coping with problems through systematic problem solving, avoiding high-risk situations through more intelligent decision making, and improving the balance of enjoyable versus obligatory activities in one's daily schedule. Relaxation training modules, included in the first edition of this text, are not included, because the preponderance of evidence does not support the effectiveness of relaxation training in preventing or reducing drinking.

The program elements covered in this chapter have a more cognitive focus than those in the preceding chapter. For this reason, some of the material is complex and may pose difficulty for clients who suffer from cognitive and memory deficits or have low education. However, the skills contained in this chapter are of value in a comprehensive rehabilitation program. We no longer recommend a particular number or sequencing of sessions for all, because rolling admissions into treatment groups are customary in many programs. However, if conducting this approach using individual treatment, the following suggestions for sequence might be used. Because temporary cognitive deficits are often seen in the early phase of recovery, it may be preferable to present the more complex cognitive restructuring skills (i.e., managing urges, problem solving, managing anger and negative thinking, and planning for emergencies) in the later phases of a treatment program. However, for clients with less impairment, some selected skills might preferably be covered early in the training sequence, despite the complexity of the material. The unit on managing urges to drink should come very early in an outpatient program for clients troubled by urges, to help them stay sober. Similarly, problem solving can help clients to cope with a variety of problems that occur in their daily lives, and it provides a framework for the therapists to structure discussion of these problems. Repetition of this framework over time while utilizing clients' own problem situations ensures that the more abstract problem-solving skills are eventually incorporated into clients' repertoires. Planning for emergencies should come last, when possible.

For each session, refer to the end of the chapter for the session's client handouts titled Reminder Sheets. These include the Practice Exercises. The Therapist Tip Sheets at the end of the chapter should be brought to sessions to ensure key points are covered.

SESSION: MANAGING URGES TO DRINK[1]

Rationale

1. Urges to drink are normal; almost anyone who stops drinking will occasionally think about starting up again. (By urges we mean desiring, wanting, craving, or even just thinking about a drink, even though you intend not to drink.) There is no problem with thinking about drinking, so long as you don't *act* on those urges. You may feel guilty about the urges (even though you have not acted on them). However, it is useful to think of urges as a warning of danger and a signal to take action. Urges are a sign that something is wrong. The purpose of this session is to teach you to identify the types of situations or events that can trigger urges, the thoughts that can be dangerous in these situations, and some ways to catch yourself so you don't actually slip. Sometimes the urges or thoughts are obvious, but sometimes they can creep up on you, almost without being noticed.

2. What are some common situations in which people may have urges to go back to drinking? (Please provide examples of your own as well.)

    a. *Remembering life as it was.* Some recovering alcoholics think about drinking as if it were some long-lost friend. For example, "I remember how good it felt when I'd take a few six-packs down to the lake and go fishing," "What's New Year's Eve without a drink?", or "A cold one sure tasted good."

    b. *Triggers in the environment.* Triggers associated with drinking are a major source of urges and include the sight of alcohol or a bar, seeing other people drink, and time cues, such as a certain time of day (getting off work) or day of the week (Friday night). When you leave a trigger situation, you may still feel urges for some time.

---

[1]This session has been adapted from Brown and Lichtenstein (1979), used by permission of the authors; from Rohsenow and Monti (1994); and from our studies of urge-specific coping skills.

c. *Crisis or stress.* During stress or crisis, an ex-drinker may say, "I *need* a drink right now. When this is all over, I'll stop drinking again." Anger is a very common trigger for drinking.

d. *Feeling uncomfortable about being sober.* Some people find that new problems arise because of being sober, and they desire to drink to end those new problems. For example, "I'm being very short-tempered and irritable around my family. Maybe it's more important for me to be a good-natured parent and spouse than it is for me to stop drinking right now," or "I'm no fun to be around when I'm not drinking. I don't think I should stop drinking, because if I do, people won't enjoy or like me as much."

e. *Testing control.* Sometimes, after a period of successful sobriety, ex-drinkers become overconfident. For example, "I bet I can have a few drinks with the guys tonight and go back on the wagon tomorrow morning," "I bet I can have just one drink," or "Let's see if I can leave a six-pack in the refrigerator, just for guests, without drinking."

f. *Self-doubts.* You may doubt your ability to succeed at things. For example, "I just have no willpower," or "I tried to quit many times before and none of those efforts worked out; why should I expect this one to last?"

It is often difficult for clients to grasp the material on analyzing and changing thoughts. Introducing the concept of cognitive analysis and restructuring can be particularly difficult for alcoholics in treatment. If the concept is not understood from the outset, then many of the benefits of cognitive coping skills can be lost.

Clients may initially be unaware of the thoughts and feelings that precede the decision to have a drink. They may simply state that they are not aware of any thought/feeling triggers, and that they "just start drinking, and that's all." This lack of awareness makes it difficult for clients to initiate the use of appropriate coping skills.

It helps first to explore the trigger situations in which these urges and thoughts occurred. Then, the idea of "slowing down the action" (as in an instant replay on TV or a slow-motion film sequence) is useful. Spend time helping clients become aware of these "automatic thoughts" or beliefs they must have had about the situation that led to the feelings. When clients feel comfortable examining the chain of thoughts associated with a previous urge to drink or relapse, the notions of self-monitoring (or self-awareness) and of modifying one's thoughts (cognitive restructuring) can then be more readily introduced. The primary goal is to gradually make clients more aware of their thought processes when they have an urge to drink, and of their ability to control or counteract these thoughts with more adaptive coping thoughts that promote abstinence. For clients who continue to have trouble grasping cognitive methods, focus more on the behavioral methods of combating urges.

---

3. Try to identify your own specific negative thoughts and excuses for drinking. What thoughts about alcohol preceded your last drinking episode after a period of sobriety? Which thoughts about alcohol seem to be associated with the most frequent or strongest

urges to drink? What circumstances, people, or events trigger these urges? On the board, list these under column headings: Triggers, Thoughts about Drinking, Feelings and Urges, Behavior.

Skill Guidelines

1. *Change the trigger situation.* Think about what event or situation is triggering your urge to drink. Then think about how to change or prevent these triggers. Some ways to change the triggers include:

    a. *Plan ahead to prevent avoidable triggers.* Don't go to parties or restaurants where alcohol is served. Plan sober activities for Friday and Saturday nights, if those times are triggers.

    b. *Escape the situation.* If you find yourself in a situation that gives you an urge, leave; go to a safe place or person, then use your skills to bring your urge down. After leaving many situations, especially conflicts, your urge will continue for awhile, so it is important to learn how to change your thoughts about drinking, also.

2. *Change your thoughts about drinking.* You will need to learn how to cope with your urges to drink, whether you leave the situation or not. Here are some ways to cope with urges by managing thoughts about drinking:

    a. *Challenge them.* Use other thoughts to challenge the thoughts that would lead to drinking. For example, "I *can't* have just one drink and then stop," "Is it worth the risk to test myself? If I fail the test, I lose everything I gained and have to start over," or "I don't have to drink to unwind after work; I can watch TV or take a walk instead," or "I can still have good times without drinking. It may feel a little strange at first, but in time, I will feel more comfortable."

    b. *Think about all the benefits of sobriety.* Thoughts about the positive consequences of sobriety that you personally expect can help to weaken your urge to drink. Make your own personal list of positive consequences, such as better physical health, improved family life, setting a good example for your kids, greater job stability, more money available for recreation and paying bills, increased self-respect and respect from others, and so on. When you have an urge, it helps to think about these positive consequences of sobriety. You might carry a card listing the benefits of sobriety and look at it whenever you catch yourself thinking about drinking. Put an asterisk by the positive consequences that matter most to you.

    c. *Think about the negative consequences of relapse.* It also can help to remind yourself of what you would lose if you went back to drinking. This can be different from losses in the past. Instead, think about what you would lose in the future if you returned to drinking. Try to conjure up an image of a specific unpleasant consequence of drinking. Make a list of the negative consequences of returning to drinking on the reverse side of the card that lists the benefits of sobriety, and put an asterisk by the ones that matter most to you. At moments of temptation, think about the consequences or take out the card and read it over slowly three or four times. You can counteract urges to drink by thinking about the "cons" of drinking and the "pros" of sobriety.

3. *Delay the decision.* When you have an urge to drink, put off the decision to drink for 15 minutes. Most urges go away if you do not drink; they do not remain as strong after a little time has passed. Remind yourself that the urge will decrease in strength if you just wait awhile.

4. *Do something else.* Find some activity that you could do immediately that will take your mind off drinking. Distracting activities can be pleasurable (such as shooting hoops or watching a video) or involve a sense of accomplishment and satisfaction (such as getting the bills paid or the shopping done). When urges are particularly strong or persistent, it helps to involve a sober person as a support in the activity, ranging from simply socializing with sober friends to talking it over with your sponsor. These activities should occur in a safe place (e.g., don't go bowling at a place that serves beer) and occupy your mind enough that you will be distracted from the urges. Once you are involved in another activity, urges are likely to decrease rapidly.

5. *Sober support.* Call someone who, in the past, has been helpful talking you through problems or urges to drink. It is important that the person be really helpful. Consider individuals such as your AA sponsor or a sober friend.

Exercise in Group

Use the coping techniques listed under Skill Guidelines to help group members develop individualized strategies they can employ to combat craving. Link these strategies to the triggers and thoughts generated earlier by the group during discussion of point 3 of the Rationale. Although this session does not include any explicit modeling or role playing, clients can be asked to imagine a difficult, high-risk situation as vividly as possible, describe it, and then practice coping with the thoughts and craving, using some of the methods in the Skill Guidelines.

Introducing the Practice Exercise

Ask clients to write out lists of (1) personal benefits of staying sober, and (2) negative consequences that would likely occur if they returned to drinking. Distribute 3" × 5" cards and instruct group members to transfer their completed lists onto them, in accordance with the suggestion in points 2 and 3 of the Skill Guidelines.

SESSION: PROBLEM SOLVING

Rationale

1. People often find themselves confronted by difficult situations. A situation becomes a problem if the person has no effective coping response immediately available to handle it.

2. Problems are part of everyday life. They arise in dealings with other people (e.g., handling social situations, feelings about others), and from your own thoughts and emotions (e.g., the way you look at a situation, self-critical thoughts, desires for the future). Think of examples from among the problems you have described in previous sessions.

3. Effective problem solving requires recognizing that you face a problem situation and resisting the temptations either to respond impulsively or to "do nothing." Coming up with an effective solution requires that you pause to assess the situation, so that you can decide which actions will be in your own best interest.

4. Sometimes the problem situation may involve wanting to drink, such as at a party. At other times, the problem itself may not involve drinking, but your tendency may be to act impulsively to find a quick and easy solution. If you don't find a good solution, then the problem can build up over time, and the pressure may eventually get to you and trigger drinking. Drinking may appear to be an easy way out. Effective problem-solving strategies must therefore be a part of everyone's program for sobriety, because problems can easily set the stage for a relapse.

Skill Guidelines[2]

1. *Problem recognition.* (This element was adapted from Intagliata, 1979.) Ask yourself, "Is there a problem?" The first task is to recognize that a problem exists. What are some of the clues that indicate that there is a problem?
   a. Clues you get from your bodies (e.g., indigestion, craving).
   b. Clues you get from your thoughts and feelings (e.g., urges to drink or feelings of anxiety, depression, loneliness, and fear).
   c. Clues you get from your behavior (worse performance at work, dealing poorly with your family or friends, not taking care of your appearance, etc.).
   d. Clues you get from noticing the way you react to other people (e.g., anger, lack of interest, withdrawal).
   e. Clues others give you (e.g., they appear to avoid you, to criticize you).

> Problem solving is a skill that provides a flexible coping repertoire in situations that have not been previously encountered. Problem recognition is crucial, especially when the impulse is to minimize or deny problems. The very act of analyzing a problem situation and coming up with a range of possible solutions can also be a direct form of coping that can be used as an alternative to drinking when one is faced with a difficult situation. Situations requiring solutions can be alcohol-specific (e.g., at a party where drinks are available), general (e.g., family illness, conflict at work), intrapersonal (e.g., feeling confused, lonely, depressed, tense), or interpersonal (e.g., family argument).
>
> Training in problem solving is used to accelerate the process of developing higher-order coping strategies that go beyond situation-specific skills. This enhances generalization of coping skills beyond the treatment situation and, in effect, encourages clients to "become their own therapists" when they are on their own.

---

[2]The overall problem-solving approach is adapted from D'Zurilla and Goldfried (1971).

2. *Identify the problem.* Ask yourself, "What is the problem?" Having recognized that something is wrong, try to identify the problem as precisely as possible. Gather as much information and as many facts as you can to help clarify the problem. Be concrete and define the problem in terms of behavior, whenever possible. Try to break it down into specific parts; you may find it easier to manage each of the parts than to confront the entire problem all at once.

3. *Consider various approaches.* (This element is adapted from Bedell, Archer, & Marlowe, 1980.) Ask yourself, "What can I do?" It is important to develop a number of solutions to a given problem, because the first one that comes to mind may not be the best. The following methods will help you to identify several approaches that could be useful in solving a problem, so that you will be more likely to settle on a good solution and implement it effectively:

   a. *Brainstorming.* Generate solutions without stopping to evaluate whether the ideas are good or bad. It is more helpful to write them down, so that you can review them when deciding which one to try. Write down all the ideas you get; do not stop to evaluate whether they are good or bad. More is better. This helps you get all your ideas out into the open, so you can decide how well they solve your problem, without rejecting any of them too hastily.

   b. *Change your point of view or frame of reference.* It helps to step back and get a little distance from the situation. Imagine that you are advising a friend about what to do. A different perspective may help you generate more alternative solutions or change your attitude toward the problem.

   c. *Adapt a solution that has worked before.* Perhaps you can think of a solution that worked well for you in a similar situation, or ask someone else about solutions that have worked for them in the past. An old solution will probably have to be modified to fit your present needs, but it can give you a good starting point.

4. *Select the most promising approach.* Think ahead. Ask yourself, "What will happen if . . . ?" Identify the most probable outcomes for each possible approach; be sure to include both positive and negative outcomes, both long- and short-term consequences. Consider what factors in your life may be used as resources to help you implement each approach, and what factors may interfere. Arrange all the potential solutions according to their consequences and desirability. The solution that maximizes positive consequences and minimizes negative ones is the one to implement first.

5. *Assess the effectiveness of the selected approach.* Implement your decision. Ask yourself, "How did it work?" Remember that the solution may not be immediate—you may have to keep working at it. Evaluate the strengths and weaknesses of your plan as you proceed by asking yourself, "What difficulties am I encountering? Am I getting the results I expected? Can I do something to make this approach more effective?" If, after you give the plan a fair chance, it doesn't seem to be resolving the problem, move on to the second-choice solution and follow the same procedure.

Behavior Rehearsal Role Plays

Clients should work through the problem recognition stage to identify problems on which they would like to work. Select one at a time, have the client describe it as accurately as possible, and have the whole group brainstorm solutions, which should be listed on the black-

board. Then, have the group reason through the process of weighing the alternatives to select the most promising one. Have them articulate both advantages and disadvantages for
every alternative as a means of combating black-and-white thinking. Prioritize the alternatives. If it seems appropriate, role-play and evaluate the effectiveness of the most promising
one(s).

If clients have difficulty coming up with appropriate problems to work on, present the
following hypothetical problem to the group:

> Your landlord is always crabby when he comes to collect the rent. One of the windows
> in your bedroom was cracked when you moved in; during a cold night, it cracked all
> the way, and a section is now out. When the landlord comes to collect the rent, you
> mention it to him. He screams at you and accuses you of breaking the window, saying
> that it was never cracked. Whenever he was crabby before, you simply let it go, but this
> time, he says you must pay to have the window replaced.

Present various definitions of the problem and have clients select the best one:

> The problem is that your landlord is a real grouch.
> The problem is that his screaming has made you feel real down and hurt.
> The problem is that you don't have enough money to pay for a new window.
> The problem is that your window is cracked and should be repaired by the landlord.
>   (Correct)

Consider various approaches to solving the problem and have clients select the most promising one. Demonstrate the brainstorming process and the factors that go into selecting the
apparent best solution.

Refer to the end of the chapter for the Reminder Sheet and Practice Exercise for this
session.

Introducing the Practice Exercise

This exercise asks clients to identify a difficult problem they have and to brainstorm a list
of possible approaches to solving the problem.

SESSION: INCREASING PLEASANT ACTIVITIES

Rationale

1. This session focuses on the role of pleasant activities in developing a sober lifestyle.
"Lifestyle" is a word that describes the usual pattern of one's day-to-day activities.

2. Many alcoholics feel a void in their lives after they stop drinking. If you had a life
composed of eating, sleeping, working, and drinking, and then you stopped drinking,
you're left with just eating, sleeping, and working. For many alcoholics, all recreational and
social activities included drinking, so avoiding alcohol means giving up all friends and past
ways of having fun. The absence of pleasant leisure activities can be a major problem.

3. The more a person engages in pleasant activities, the more positive his/her feelings.

Likewise, the fewer pleasant activities, the more likely it is that negative feelings such as boredom, loneliness, and depression will occur. This suggests that pleasant leisure-time activities may be a powerful tool for preventing or controlling these negative feelings.

4. Many people spend most of their time meeting obligations that are not necessarily pleasant, but that must be performed (e.g., a job, housework, yardwork, errands)—things they "should" do rather than things they "want to" do. If your lifestyle is full of "shoulds" and totally lacking in "want to's," you may start to believe that you "owe" yourself a drink or drug as a reward for working so hard. It is best to achieve some balance between activities you should do and those you want to do (Marlatt & Gordon, 1985).

Skill Guidelines

1. *Develop a menu of pleasant activities.* The first step in changing your lifestyle is to target some pleasant activities that you want to initiate or increase in frequency. One way to do that is to brainstorm a list of activities and pick out some activities that are pleasant for you. People are very different with respect to the specific kinds of activities they experience as pleasant. Let's now brainstorm the activities that you personally find pleasant. Then, let's write down the ones that are not associated with your drinking. This list forms a "menu" of pleasant activities. Some of the pleasant activities may be things you used to enjoy but haven't done in a long time. Other items on your menu may be things you have wanted to do but never got around to trying.

2. Some pleasant activities can become "positive addictions" (Glasser, 1976). If a negative addiction (e.g., alcohol) can be described as an activity that feels good at first but results in feeling bad later on and causes harm in the long run, a positive addiction (e.g., jogging) is an activity that may not feel so good at first but becomes more desirable as time goes on and is very beneficial in the long run. A positive addiction is an activity that meets the following criteria: (a) It is noncompetitive; (b) it does not depend on others; (c) it has some value for you (physical, mental, or spiritual); (d) you can improve with practice (but you are the only one who is aware of your progress); and (e) you accept your level of performance without criticizing yourself. Examples include relaxation, meditation, exercise (jogging, swimming, skiing, cycling, etc.), hobbies, reading, cultural activities, and creative skills (music, art, writing, etc.).

3. The next step after completing your menu is to *develop a pleasant activities plan.* Try scheduling a small block of time each day (30–60 minutes) for pleasant activities. Begin this "personal time" by sitting quietly and mentally reviewing your menu of pleasant activities. You probably will not want to do the same thing every day. One day, you may feel the need for relaxation, another day, for exercise, and yet another day for gardening or music. Schedule some time each day, but do not schedule the activity, so that what you do in your personal time does not become another obligation.

4. As a group, let's discuss the following strategies for, and obstacles to, increasing one's rate of pleasant activities (adapted from Lewinsohn, Antonuccio, Steinmetz, & Teri, 1984):

> a. *Commitment.* Putting a pleasant activities plan into action requires a strong commitment. You must be willing to establish priorities and perhaps also rearrange other activities in your life.

b. *Balance.* The goal is to achieve an adequate balance between the activities you "should" do and the activities you "want" to do. Note that balance is not the same as equality: There will likely be more "shoulds" than "want to's." "Balance" refers to each individual's degree of satisfaction with his/her daily life.

c. *Planning.* What problems or circumstances might interfere with your completing your plan? How will you take care of competing demands on your time?

d. *Pleasantness.* Be sure to choose activities that you find highly enjoyable.

e. *Anxiety.* Anxiety can interfere with your engaging in or enjoying pleasant activities. This may dissipate with time, or you may need to choose other activities.

f. *Control.* If you stick to your plan, you will achieve a measure of control over your daily schedule. You will also add some activities that you find enjoyable and rewarding.

Introducing the Practice Exercise

This assignment asks group members to write out a personal list of pleasant activities that are not associated with drinking for them. They should also make appointments with themselves for "personal time." *After* their personal time, they should record their activities.

SESSION: ANGER MANAGEMENT

Rationale

1. Anger or irritation is a normal human emotion. It occurs when:
   a. Things seem out of our control.
   b. We think our rights have been stepped on.
   c. We are not getting what we want or what we think is right.

> Many alcoholics don't like to use the word "anger" for lower levels of anger. Rather than insisting on the term, try "irritation" or another, similar term. Use the term they agree to throughout, instead of "anger."

2. There is a distinction between anger as a *feeling (emotion)* and some of the behavioral *consequences* of anger, such as aggression, impulsive actions, passivity, and passive–aggressive behavior. Some of these consequences increase the likelihood of drinking. Anger itself is neither good nor bad. It can be an intense feeling, and the reaction to that feeling may be constructive or destructive.

Destructive effects:
a. Anger causes mental confusion. It leads to impulsive actions and poor decision making, including drinking.
b. Aggressive reactions to anger decrease effective communication, create emotional distance, and trigger hostility in others. Can you think of some examples in your life of how aggressive behavior has backfired?

c. Passive reactions to anger leave you feeling helpless or depressed, reduce self-esteem, mask real feelings with an appearance of indifference, are a barrier to communication, and build resentments that may spill out at the slightest provocation in a tantrum or drinking.

Constructive effects:

a. Feelings of anger let you know that there is a problematic situation and energize you to resolve it. Use anger as a signal that there is a problem that needs solving.

b. An assertive response to anger increases your personal power over unpleasant situations, helps you communicate your negative feelings and their intensity, can be used to change destructive aspects of a relationship, helps you avoid future misunderstandings, and may strengthen a relationship. An effective response with appropriate assertiveness helps you to increase the constructive effects and decrease the destructive effects of angry feelings.

3. Relationship between anger and problem drinking: Studies of people who relapsed after alcoholism treatment have revealed that many took their first drink when they were angry or upset. Anger seems to make people highly vulnerable to relapse. Therefore, it is particularly important to learn to cope with anger and irritation in a constructive way.

Skill Guidelines

Most emotions are best understood by using a behavior chain. Anger does not just happen. People often think that situations or events make them angry, but actually it is their thoughts or beliefs about the trigger situations or events that result in anger. Let's show what we mean by putting a behavior chain on the board to show how alternative thoughts affect feelings.

Trigger	→ Thoughts/beliefs	→ Feelings →	Behavior
Driver cuts in front of you	"That S.O.B. How dare he!"	Fury	Dangerous driving
Driver cuts in front of you	"He must be in a hurry, maybe late to work."	Calm	Safe driving

The first step to managing your anger is to become more aware of your personal triggers and thoughts about those triggers. Increased awareness can help you to identify angry feelings early, before they grow and get out of hand, to change the thoughts that aggravate anger, and to change your behavior in response to the anger.

1. Become more aware of situations that trigger anger.
   a. *Direct triggers*: a direct attack on you, whether verbal (e.g., insult) or nonverbal (e.g., physical attack, obscene gesture), or frustration resulting from inability to reach a goal (e.g., your ex-wife won't let you see the kids).

    b. *Indirect triggers*: observing an attack on someone else, or your appraisal of a situation (e.g., feeling that you are being blamed, thinking that someone is disapproving of you, or feeling that too many demands are being made of you).

2. Become more aware of your automatic thoughts associated with anger.

This is the hardest step at first. Often, these thoughts occur so automatically and quickly that we are not aware of them. Sometimes you may notice the words that are running through your head, such as "That crazy loon, I'm not going to let him get away with that!" Other times, you can figure out what thoughts or beliefs you must be having in order to produce the emotion. For example, you say "Hi" to a friend and he just grunts and walks on:

Thoughts	Feelings
"Uh oh, he must be annoyed with me about something. What did I do to make him mad?"	Fear Guilt
"How dare he! After all I've done for him!"	Irritation Anger
"Poor guy. His boss must be ragging on him again."	Sympathy Calm

3. Change your thoughts about the trigger.
    a. The first thing to do is *calm down.* As long as you keep cool, *you* will be in control of the situation. Here are some phrases to help you cool off in a crisis:

"Slow down."	"Chill out."
"Take it easy."	"Easy does it."
"Take a deep breath."	"Relax."
"Cool it."	"Count to 10."

       Decide on one or two phrases like these that you can say to yourself to help you cool your anger while in the situation.

    b. After you've slowed yourself down, think about the situation: "What's getting me angry?" Question your interpretation of the situation. Think about whether your reaction was realistic: "Is it really that bad?", "Am I overreacting?", "Is it really worth getting stressed out over this little thing?"

    c. Think about whether there might be another interpretation of the situation: "Maybe she's not trying to control me, she's just trying to help," "Maybe my son's not mad at me. He's scared that I might start drinking again," or "Is this really an attack or insult?"

    d. Think about the negative consequences of getting angry: "If I blow up, I risk my sobriety," "If I yell, I'll just make things worse," or "If I stay cool, I'll handle this better."

    e. Replace the negative thoughts with more positive thoughts: "There are a lot of jerks in the world but so what? I don't have to let them bother me," "Life's too short to sweat the small stuff," "This will be over soon. I can handle it," or "He's not trying to put me down, he's just upset about something I did that was wrong. Let me fix this."

4. Change what you do in response to the trigger.
   a. Think about your options: "What is in my best interests here? My anger should be a signal that it's time to do some problem solving," or "What can I do? What is the best thing for me to do?" (Communications skills, or other coping skills might be used in this situation.)
   b. Choose possible behaviors that will make you calmer or will solve the problem:

   > Leave the situation (useful with strangers, impersonal events).
   > Take time out to cool.
   > Use assertiveness to request a change.
   > Analyze how to solve or cope with the problem.
   > Talk to the person about it in a calm, rational way.

   c. After trying to resolve the problem, you may find that you cannot resolve the conflict, and you still feel angry. Remember that you can't fix everything. Thinking about it over and over again only makes you more upset. Try to shake it off—it may not be so serious. Don't let it interfere with your life. Some actions you can take include the following:

   > Call a sober friend to help you calm down.
   > Plan something fun to counteract the lousy feelings.

Modeling (Optional)

The therapists present the clients with the following scenario:

> Your spouse (or friend, or teenage child) is helping you to wash and wax your car. In the middle of the job, he/she suddenly walks away, goes inside, and turns on the TV. You find yourself increasingly angry as you look at the work that remains and the mess that has to be cleaned up. You decide to confront your work partner.

The therapists should demonstrate an appropriate response to this situation, articulating their self-statements for anger management aloud:

> Cool-down phrases ("OK, chill down and think a minute.").
> Thoughts about the situation ("What's getting me angry? Is this a personal attack? Am I expecting too much?").
> Thoughts about options ("What is in my best interest here? What can I do?").

Behavior Rehearsal Role Plays

Have clients each list a trigger situation and the thoughts or beliefs they each had in the situation that led to anger. Guide the group in generating positive, alternative thoughts and behaviors in each situation. Then, have clients discuss what they think the consequences of these alternatives would be.

Introducing the Practice Exercise

This assignment asks clients to practice using these skills in an anger-provoking situation. Clients describe the situation, calming phrases, anger-increasing thoughts, alternative anger-reducing thoughts, and behaviors to solve the problem or to calm themselves.

SESSION: MANAGING NEGATIVE THINKING

Rationale

1. Negative moods, such as depression, tension, guilt, and loneliness, can set the stage for drinking. Often, these moods result from the way we think. Many times, we assume a negative thinking style about events that could just as easily be interpreted as neutral or even positive.

2. Thinking negatively can lead to all sorts of negative emotions and tension, which can then lead to drinking as an escape. For example, "My boss must really hate me for being unreliable, so there is no chance he will ever promote me. I may as well stop trying to do such a good job, or perhaps I should just quit work."

3. Negative thinking can become a self-fulfilling prophecy, leading to chronic low self-respect, anger, depression, fatigue, stress, anxiety, or boredom. For example, if you think about giving up or quitting work, you may start slacking off and eventually get a warning or be fired. You must therefore learn to recognize your negative thoughts and moods as signals to think about ways to change the negative thinking, rather than as signals to give up on yourself and drink. Your thoughts are sometimes called "self-talk." Negative thoughts are sometimes referred to in AA jargon as "stinking thinking."

4. Usually, changing your thinking doesn't make you feel better instantly. It takes time and practice before you learn to catch yourself thinking negatively and develop positive thinking to change your moods and feelings of self-worth. Just because you don't notice feeling much better the instant you change your thinking doesn't mean it's not working.

5. We often think that situations or events make us feel bad, when, in reality, it is our thoughts about the situations or events that determine how good or bad we feel. We use a behavior chain to show how our thoughts about events affect our feelings and behavior.

Trigger	→	Thoughts/beliefs	→	Feelings	→	Behavior
Event, situation		Negative thoughts		Feel bad		Destructive
		Positive thoughts		Feel good		Constructive

Can you think of examples from your own life that illustrate this chain of events?

Often, people feel helpless and unable to change the way they feel. They say, "I can't do anything about it. I just feel depressed and tired all the time. Leave me alone!" They seem to be saying:

Events   →   Feelings

However, it is usually negative thinking that causes the negative feelings. You *can* learn to recognize and then control or change your feelings by changing your thoughts. The thoughts that lead to negative moods/feelings are called either "negative thoughts" or negative "self-talk."

Skill Guidelines

1. The main steps to changing your negative thinking are as follows:
    a. *Catch yourself thinking negatively.* You must learn what kinds of negative thinking habits you have learned over the years and have come to use automatically. You must be able to recognize them when they occur. Your moods might be a signal. For example, if you are feeling depressed, you probably were thinking negatively just before that and didn't even know it.
    b. *Stop the negative thinking pattern* and substitute a more positive or reasonable set of thoughts; that is, challenge or replace negative thoughts with positive or neutral thoughts.

2. *Identify your negative thoughts.* Can you think of negative thoughts that might be behind some negative mood states or other common events? Start with the following easy examples:

Trigger	Thoughts	Feelings
Your kid broke a glass during breakfast.	_____ _____ _____	Angry, upset
Your boss wasn't very friendly today.	_____ _____	Tense, worried, depressed, upset

Another way to get a list of thoughts that lead to negative moods is to think about previous events that led to strong emotions or drinking. Examples of such thoughts are as follows: "I am a stupid idiot, I can't do anything right"; "He must hate me"; "Everything I do is wrong"; "If I blow this, I am a total failure"; "I should never do that"; "People are always out to get me"; "I am always letting people down"; "I must do everything perfectly and never make mistakes"; "Everyone should love me all the time." (Have group members come up with personal examples of triggers and thoughts.) It may be helpful to categorize the list of thoughts you have generated as a group. The guidelines provided by Ellis (1975) include the following categories:
    a. *Unrealistic goals* (perfectionism): I must, should, have to do everything right" or "Other people should always be reliable, trustworthy, friendly, on time."
    b. *Catastrophizing*: "If things don't work out exactly the way I expect, then it's useless, awful, terrible, the end of the world."
    c. *Overgeneralization*: "I can never be on time"; "I am always and forever going to be depressed."
    d. *Expecting the worst*: "I will never get my act together"; "This marriage is doomed

to fail"; "I know nobody really likes me"; "Even strangers won't ever like me if they get to know me."

e. *Self-put-downs*: "I don't deserve better"; "I am stupid, unreliable, weak"; "My dad always said I was no good."

f. *"Black-and-white" thinking*: Goes with perfectionism and catastrophizing. "If I am ever late for work at all, then I will get fired and never, ever get another job for as long as I live"; "If people don't totally love me, then they must hate me"; "Either I am all good or I am all bad."

3. Stop the negative thinking and replace it with more healthy, positive thinking. You may not notice it at first, but with repetition and practice, this will gradually help you to begin to feel less moody, depressed, frustrated, angry, tense, or upset, and to feel better about yourself. You can change how you think about events or people that used to bother you. For example, if someone says you are a no-good jerk, you can let that upset you. In effect, you are either saying "I agree, I am no good" or "He has no right to insult me that way." However, you can counteract the negative thinking with a more positive thought: "I may act like a jerk sometimes, but I am really a good person who is trying very hard to be better," or "He's right that I did one dumb thing, but it doesn't mean that I am a total jerk forever."

To summarize, there are four steps in changing negative thinking:

a. Stop and become aware of what you are thinking.

b. Question the thoughts: "Are these thoughts valid or am I jumping to conclusions?", "Did I interpret the situation correctly?", "Am I overreacting?", "Is this stinking thinking?"

c. Replace the thoughts with more positive thoughts: "It's not true that I can't do anything right. I just didn't do this thing right," "It's not true that sobriety will never get any easier. Just take it one day at a time," "Don't sweat the small stuff. This won't matter in the long run."

d. Afterwards, change your behavior. After your thinking has become more positive, develop a plan to solve the problem, if possible.

4. Work through some examples on the board with the group. Use the example below or develop your own group's examples. List *some* of the positive alternative thoughts, and have the group generate more.

Trigger Event

It's your first week on a new job. You miss the morning bus that you take to work because you misread the bus schedule. You will be late to work today.

Negative Thoughts

"I can't do anything right."

"I must be really stupid if I made a mistake with a simple bus schedule."

"Now my boss will think I'm an irresponsible person."

"I wanted to be really good (perfect) on the job, and now this ruins it all."

"I'll probably get fired for being late. How will I ever pay the bills now? I will never find a new job."

"The boss knows I'm a recovering alcoholic, and he'll think I've been drinking again."

"Life isn't fair. Just when things start going good for me, something always happens to mess it all up.

Negative Feelings

Scared, depressed, angry, anxious, worried, tense.

Strong desire or urge to drink.

Consequence: Arrive at work feeling defensive, incompetent, and unable to focus on what to do.

Positive Alternative Thoughts

"Darn, I missed the bus. Well, don't get all upset about it. It won't do any good and will just get me thinking about booze."

"Nobody's perfect. Anyone could misread a bus schedule once in a while."

"I'd rather not be late, but if I am, it's not the end of the world."

"When I start to feel upset like this, that's my signal to stop, take a deep breath, relax, and think positive. What can I do about the situation right now?"

"I can call the boss and let him know that I'm late and on my way. He'll probably appreciate my letting him know and won't have to wonder where I am."

"Even if my boss *is* a little angry at me, I've got plenty more days to show him that I'm a good worker. He'll get over it as soon as he sees that I'm usually reliable."

"I'm proud of myself for not flying to pieces over this the way I would have in the past."

Positive Feelings

Calm, confident, hopeful, more relaxed.

Feels in control of thoughts.

No urge to drink.

Consequence: Appears calm at work, did not set up a vicious negative cycle.

After group discussion of personal examples of how to change negative thinking into positive thinking, remind the group members that this is really a simple, three-step process:
- Catch yourself thinking negatively as soon as possible, before you get too upset or want to drink.
- *Stop* yourself. Become aware of the negative thoughts. Interrupt or break the chain of negative thoughts.
- Challenge the negative thoughts and substitute positive, more reasonable thinking.

5. *Categories of positive thoughts that counteract negative thinking.* Most specific, positive self-talk falls into a few general categories. If clients are aware of these basic types, they may be better able to come up with positive statements for any given situation. (If you do

not wish to cover all this in one session, just choose the most relevant categories for the group.)

a. *Recalling good things about life and about yourself.* For instance, remind yourself about what went well today, or what things you usually do well. What's good about you as a person? What do you enjoy? What nice things has another person done for you?

b. *Challenging irrational beliefs and unrealistic expectations.* You can recognize these because they usually contain extreme words such as the following:
   • Should, must, ought, have to
   • Awful, terrible, disastrous
   • Always, never, no one, everyone

   For example, compare "Others should always love and approve of what I do, and if they don't, then it is terrible" with "It's nice to have love and approval from others, but even without it I can still enjoy and accept myself."

c. *Decatastrophizing.* Often, negative emotions are the result of predicting catastrophic consequences. These thoughts can be defused by examining the probability of the feared event, its degree of unpleasantness, your ability to prevent it from occurring, and your ability to accept and deal with the worst possible outcome.

d. *Relabeling the distress.* Tell yourself that the anxiety, frustration, or anger is a signal to use your coping skills rather than to get upset and drink. For example, physical pain can be an important signal that there is a problem needing treatment to prevent the problem from getting worse. Although pain is uncomfortable, it alerts us to take constructive action, so it should not be ignored. Similarly, feelings of emotional distress, though uncomfortable, are important signals that the situation and your thoughts or actions may need constructive change. In the past, you may have drunk or done other destructive things to cope with your feelings, with the result that things got even worse. Thus, relabeling distress as a valuable signal telling you to cope (and no longer viewing distress as a signal to give up, or drink) is a very positive step.

e. *"Hopefulness" statements.* Often, pessimism or optimism become self-fulfilling prophecies. Making positive self-statements and giving yourself encouragement may lead to positive outcomes. For example, "I can change how I'm responding"; "I can handle this"; "I can have an effect on the situation"; "It'll probably turn out well in the long run, even though it's difficult now."

f. *Blaming the event, not yourself.* Making one mistake does not make you a dumb *person.* Everyone is human and makes mistakes sometimes. Blame the *event* or *behavior* only—not yourself as a person, and not for all time, just for that once.

g. *Reminding yourself to stay "on task."* Focus on what needs to be done. For example, "Don't think about being upset; just relax and think about what you have to do." You can't change the past but you can change what you do in the future.

h. *Self-reinforcement.* When you've handled a difficult situation well, tell yourself so— pat yourself on the back with your positive thoughts. For example: "I started off really upset about Jim being late for our appointment, but I did a pretty good job of calming myself down. I'm proud of myself for bringing my feelings back to a manageable level."

Exercise in Group

Ask a group member to share a recent experience that he/she found upsetting in some way. Ask him/her to describe the situation, his/her reaction to it, and negative thinking about it. Then encourage the group to work with the group member to generate more positive self-statements with which to handle the situation.

Introducing the Practice Exercise

Ask clients to write down one or two events in which they felt bad and to (1) identify the negative thoughts, then (2) list alternative thoughts that challenge or counteract the negative thoughts.

SESSION: SEEMINGLY IRRELEVANT DECISIONS

Rationale[3]

1. Many of the ordinary, mundane choices that you make every day seem to have nothing at all to do with drinking. Although they may not involve making a direct choice of whether to drink, they may move you, one small step at a time, closer to a confrontation with that choice. Through a series of minor decisions, you may gradually work your way closer to the point at which drinking becomes very likely. These seemingly unimportant decisions that may in fact put you on the road to drinking are called "seemingly irrelevant decisions" (SIDs).

2. People often think of themselves as victims: "Things just seemed to happen in such a way that I ended up in a high-risk situation and then had a drink. I couldn't help it." They don't recognize how perhaps dozens of their "little" decisions over a period of time gradually brought them closer and closer to their predicament. It's relatively easy to play "Monday morning quarterback" with these decisions and see how you set yourself up for relapse, but it's much harder to recognize when you are actually in the midst of the decision-making process, because so many choices don't actually seem to involve drinking at the time. Each choice you make may only take you just a little bit closer to having to make that big choice. But when alcohol isn't on your mind, it's hard to make the connection between drinking and a minor decision that seems very far removed from drinking.

3. The best solution is to think about every choice you have to make, no matter how seemingly irrelevant it is to drinking. By *thinking ahead* about each possible option you have and where it may lead, you can anticipate dangers that may lie along certain paths. It may feel awkward at first to have to consider everything so carefully, but after a while, it becomes second nature and happens automatically, without much effort. The increased control you will gain over your own sobriety is well worth the initial effort you will have to make.

4. When faced with a decision, you should generally choose a low-risk option, to avoid

---

[3]This section is adapted from Marlatt (1985a, pp. 271–274). Copyright 1985 by The Guilford Press. Adapted by permission.

putting yourself in a risky situation. On the other hand, you may for some reason decide to select a high-risk option. If you make this choice, you must also plan how to protect yourself in the high-risk situation.

5. To illustrate how some seemingly minor decisions can lead to a relapse, one client called "Stu" (not his real name) had been treated for alcohol dependence. His alcohol use had caused him numerous marital and financial problems. When asked to describe his most recent relapse, he said, "There's not much to tell. I quit drinking for 6 months, but then I was in the Shamrock Bar and began drinking again." Obviously, a bar is a high-risk locale for anyone trying to stay sober. When asked to describe what led up to his arrival in the bar, he told the following story:

> "I was going to pick up my wife after work at Denny's. But as I got close to down-town Providence, I got restless and decided to detour through downtown to see the progress on the new construction. I had left a half-hour early, so I had extra time to kill, and there was no sense getting there too early. Once I got downtown, I couldn't resist driving by the Shamrock, where I used to drink. I figured I'd park near there and walk over to the construction site. However, I needed change for the parking meter, so I went into the Shamrock to get change for a buck. After all, convenience stores won't give you change. When I walked in, I saw Hank. It would have been rude to walk out without talking with him after all this time, so I sat at his table. Before I could tell him otherwise, he'd bought me a beer, and it wouldn't have been right to refuse it. I'd been sober so long, I knew I could handle one. My wife had to bail me out of the drunk tank."

Did Stu plan his own relapse? He strongly denied any *conscious* plan to resume drinking. Yet he made a number of seemingly irrelevant decisions that led up to sitting in a bar with a drink in front of him—an extremely high-risk relapse situation. Can you identify some of these decisions? They did not appear to be drinking decisions, but were rather decisions to leave on an errand a half hour early, to detour downtown, to park in front of a bar, to get change for parking, to stay and talk with a drinker, and not to tell his friend he could not drink. In each SID, however, one of the available choices brought Stu one step closer to a high-risk situation in which relapse was all but inevitable.

6. By becoming aware of SIDs, you may be better able to take corrective action to avoid high-risk situations. It is usually much easier to decide to *avoid* a high-risk situation than to resist temptation once you are in the midst of it. For example, it would have been easier for Sam not to detour through downtown than to decide not to drink once he was in the bar.

Group Discussion

The following are examples of SID situations that have set up some recovering alcoholics for a relapse, and some examples of healthy, alternative decisions; discuss the consequences of each:

> Keeping liquor in the house for guests.
> Going to bars to see old drinking friends, watch a sporting event on TV, play darts, eat a meal, or the like.

Going to a party where people are drinking.

Keeping it a secret from your friends that you have quit drinking.

Deciding where to go to get a snack (e.g., to a liquor store or to a gas station).

Deciding what route to take when driving (to go past a favorite bar, liquor store, etc., or to detour to avoid these).

Taking a job as a bartender, in a liquor store, and so on.

Not making plans for the weekend.

Telling a friend that you have quit drinking.

Planning how to spend free time after work.

Starting conversations with people at AA or NA meetings.

Asking housemate not to bring alcohol into the house.

Describe examples of your own SIDs and how they might eventually lead to a relapse.

Exercise in Group

Ask clients to think about their last slip or relapse after a period of abstinence, and to describe the situation and events that preceded it. What decisions led up to the relapse situation? List decisions on the blackboard. After a relapse, it is easy to play "Monday morning quarterback." By becoming aware of SIDs, clients should be able to set themselves up for sobriety.

Introducing the Practice Exercise

Today's assignment asks clients to identify SIDs among recent and upcoming decisions. Make the point that clients do not necessarily have to choose the "safe" alternative, but they should at least be *aware* that their choice may ultimately lead to a high-risk relapse situation, so that they may make preparations to cope with it effectively.

SESSION: PLANNING FOR EMERGENCIES

Rationale

1. It is important to plan how to handle crisis situations on your own.

2. Major life events and life changes can be very disruptive and lead to a relapse to drinking. Some such life events might include the following:

- Social separations (e.g., divorce, death, child leaving home, close friend moving away)
- Health problems
- New responsibilities
- Adjustments to new situations
- Work-related events (e.g., losing a job, getting a new job, promotion)
- Financial changes

Can you think of other major events to add to this list?

3. Life events do not necessarily have to be negative to lead up to a relapse. Positive life

changes can also pose a risk—for example, marriage, moving, promotion, or graduation. These events may leave you feeling "on top of the world" and perhaps a little *too* confident, or may involve new, stressful responsibilities.

4. Major events in the lives of those close to you can also affect you. Family members or close friends may become upset or preoccupied with their concerns, or may begin to act differently toward you.

5. Describe a life event or life change that you can anticipate. As a group, list these on the blackboard. Consider how your event will affect your behavior and interactions with others.

Skill Guidelines

1. The major life events listed on the blackboard can be considered high-risk situations that may increase the likelihood of a relapse. What specific strategies can you use to cope with these situations? Draw on skills discussed in previous sessions, such as problem solving, decision making, managing thoughts about drinking, anger management, mood management of negative thinking and feelings, and increasing pleasant events.

2. Begin to prepare a general emergency plan for coping with a number of possible stressful situations that may arise unexpectedly. Include problem-solving skills, calling people for support, increasing attendance at AA or NA meetings, and cognitive strategies. These are only a few examples; you should provide as much specific detail as possible (e.g., names, phone numbers, locations of meetings).

Introducing the Practice Exercise

Have clients write out an emergency plan. Encourage group members to be specific regarding whom they will call for support, what AA meetings they will attend, and so on. When reviewing the plans that the clients develop, play "devil's advocate" by challenging some of them, or suggesting that one of their options does not work out (e.g., "What if both your support people are out of town?"). This provides an opportunity to test the range, depth, and flexibility of each client's current repertoire of coping skills. If necessary, introduce some reminders of previous sessions' coping skills.

Therapist Tip Sheet: Managing Urges to Drink

POINTS FOR RATIONALE

1. Urges are normal and OK. Use them as warning of danger or a need to take action.
2. Common situations that lead to urges:
   - Memories of what it was like to drink
   - Environments associated with drinking
   - Crisis or stress
   - Feeling uncomfortable about being sober
   - Desire to test control, overconfidence
   - Self-doubts
3. What people, events, places, thoughts, and feelings give you urges?
   List on board under Triggers, Thoughts about Drinking, Feelings and Urges, Behavior.

POINTS FOR BLACKBOARD (IN CAPITALS)

<u>SKILL GUIDELINES</u>

1. CHANGE THE TRIGGER SITUATION.
   - PLAN AHEAD TO AVOID.
   - ESCAPE.
2. CHANGE THOUGHTS ABOUT DRINKING.
   - CHALLENGE THOUGHTS; question and replace them.
   - Think about BENEFITS OF SOBRIETY.
   - Think about NEGATIVE CONSEQUENCES OF RELAPSE.
3. DELAY THE DECISION to drink.
4. DO SOMETHING ELSE; distracting activity involving pleasure or accomplishment.
5. Call a SOBER SUPPORT.

Reminder Sheet: Managing Urges

Here are several ways to manage urges to drink or to use drugs:

- Change the trigger situation: Plan ahead to prevent avoidable triggers or leave the situation.
- Challenge your thoughts: Do you really *need* a drink? Will you really not have fun without a drink?
- Think of the benefits of sobriety (read list on card).
- Think of the negative consequences of relapse (read list on card).
- Carry photographs of loved ones who would be disappointed if you drank.
- Delay the decision: Remind yourself that urges decrease with time.
- Do something else: Find a safe but distracting activity that gives you pleasure or satisfaction.
- Call a sober support and try to talk it out.

PRACTICE EXERCISE

One way to cope with thoughts about drinking is to remind yourself of the benefits of not drinking, and of the unpleasant things that would happen if you returned to drinking. Use this sheet to make a list of these reminders, then transfer this list onto a pocket-sized index card. Read this card whenever you start to have thoughts about drinking or using drugs.

Benefits of sobriety: _____

_____

_____

_____

_____

_____

Unpleasant consequences of drinking: _____

_____

_____

_____

_____

_____

Therapist Tip Sheet: Problem Solving

POINTS FOR RATIONALE

1. A problem is difficult if no effective coping response is immediately available.
2. Problems are part of everyday life: dealing with people or thoughts and emotions.
3. Recognize the problem, resist impulses, resist doing nothing, pause to assess.
4. Taking an easy way out (by acting impulsively, doing nothing, or drinking) causes problems to get worse, sets the stage for relapse.

POINTS FOR BLACKBOARD (IN CAPITALS)

SKILL GUIDELINES

1. CLUES TO RECOGNIZING A PROBLEM:
   - BODY (indigestion, neckache)
   - THOUGHTS AND FEELINGS (anxiety, urges, sadness, loneliness)
   - BEHAVIOR (doing worse at work, with family; poor grooming)
   - YOUR REACTIONS TO OTHERS (anger, disinterest, withdrawal)
   - OTHERS' REACTIONS TO YOU (anger, withdrawal, criticism)
2. IDENTIFY THE PROBLEM precisely, in terms of behavior; break it into specific parts.
3. CONSIDER VARIOUS APPROACHES, possible solutions:
   - BRAINSTORMING.
   - CHANGE YOUR POINT OF VIEW.
   - ADAPT A SOLUTION THAT WORKED BEFORE.
4. CHOOSE MOST PROMISING APPROACH:
   - List all probable OUTCOMES, positive and negative, long and short term.
   - Consider RESOURCES that can help, INTERFERING FACTORS.
5. PUT INTO ACTION.
6. ASSESS HOW WELL IT WORKED:
   - Evaluate STRENGTHS AND WEAKNESSES of the plan.
   - GIVE IT A FAIR TEST, allow time for it to work.

Reminder Sheet: Problem Solving

These, in brief, are the steps of the problem-solving process:

- *Recognize that* a *problem exists.* "Is there a problem?" We get clues from our bodies, our thoughts and feelings, our behavior, our reactions to other people, and the ways that other people react to us.
- *Identify the problem.* "What is the problem?" Describe the problem as accurately as you can. Break it down into manageable parts.
- *Consider various approaches to solving the problem.* "What can I do?" Brainstorm to think of as many solutions as you can. Try taking a different point of view. Try to think of solutions that worked before, and ask other people what worked for them in similar situations.
- *Select the most promising approach.* "What will happen if . . . ?" Consider all the positive and negative aspects of each possible approach, and select the one likely to solve the problem with the least hassle.
- *Assess the effectiveness of the selected approach.* "How well did it work?" After you have given the approach a fair trial, does it seem to be working out? If not, consider what you can do to beef up the plan, or give it up and try one of the other possible approaches.

PRACTICE EXERCISE

Select a problem you expect to find difficult. Describe it accurately. Brainstorm a list of possible solutions. Evaluate the possibilities, and number them in the order of your preference.

Identify the problem: _____

_____

_____

_____

_____

Brainstorm list of possible solutions: _____

_____

_____

_____

_____

Therapist Tip Sheet: Increasing Pleasant Activities

POINTS FOR RATIONALE

1. Important part of a sober lifestyle.
2. Many drinkers feel a void in their lives after they quit drinking:
   - All recreational and social activities included alcohol.
   - Have to give up all drinking-related friends and leisure activities.
3. Increasing pleasant activities increases positive feelings, decreases negative ones.
4. Imbalanced lifestyle of too many "shoulds" and not enough "wants" can trigger relapse.

POINTS FOR BLACKBOARD (IN CAPITALS)

SKILL GUIDELINES

1. Develop your own MENU OF PLEASANT ACTIVITIES not associated with drinking.
2. Some can become POSITIVE ADDICTIONS.
3. Develop a PLEASANT ACTIVITIES PLAN: SCHEDULE TIMES for pleasure.
4. STRATEGIES AND OBSTACLES:
   a. COMMITMENT needed to change priorities, activities.
   b. BALANCE needed between "shoulds" and "wants."
   c. PLANNING to deal with obstacles, competing demands on time.
   d. PLEASANTNESS—choose highly enjoyable activities.
   e. ANXIETY at first can go away with time, or change activity.
   f. CONTROL—you will feel more control over your life when you stick with a plan.

Reminder Sheet: Increasing Pleasant Activities

- Develop a list of pleasant activities not associated with drinking.
- "Positive addictions" are activities that are noncompetitive; do not depend on others; and have some physical, mental, or spiritual value for you. You can improve your performance with practice, and you can accept your level of performance without criticizing yourself.
- Plan 30–60 minutes of "personal time" each day for pleasant activities.
- The goal is to achieve some balance between the things that you should do and the things that you want to do, so that you feel satisfied with your daily life.
- The more fun things you have to do, the less you will miss alcohol or use alcohol to create fun in your life.

PRACTICE EXERCISE

First, write down your own personal "menu" of pleasant activities that are not associated with substance use. _____

_____

_____

_____

_____

Now, schedule 30–60 minutes of "personal time" every day to engage in these activities. Set aside the time, but do not decide on the activity until the time comes. Select the activity from the menu above.

	Appointments for personal time	After your personal time, record the activity you decided to do
Monday	_____	_____
Tuesday	_____	_____
Wednesday	_____	_____
Thursday	_____	_____
Friday	_____	_____
Saturday	_____	_____
Sunday	_____	_____

Therapist Tip Sheet: Anger Management

POINTS FOR RATIONALE

1. Anger is a normal emotion when we feel out of control, rights violated, don't get what we want.
2. Distinction between *feeling (emotion)* and some *behavioral consequences*:
   - Anger or irritation as a feeling is neither good nor bad.
   - Behavioral reaction can be constructive or destructive.
3. Some consequences (aggression, impulsive actions, passivity, passive–aggression) increase likelihood of drinking.
4. Destructive effects:
   - Anger causes mental confusion, can lead to poor decisions, impulsive acts, drinking.
   - Aggressive reactions: poor communication, emotional distance, hostile response.
   - Passive reactions: feeling helpless, lower self-esteem, poor communication, resentments.

   Constructive effects:
   - Anger is a signal that there is a problem that needs solving.
   - Anger provides energy to act.
   - Assertive response: more power, better communication, improve relationships, resolve problem, avoid future misunderstandings.

POINTS FOR BLACKBOARD (IN CAPITALS)

BEHAVIOR CHAIN to show how thoughts/beliefs about triggers result in anger.

TRIGGER → THOUGHTS/BELIEFS → FEELINGS → BEHAVIOR

SKILL GUIDELINES

1. BECOME AWARE OF TRIGGERS—situations that trigger anger:
   - DIRECT TRIGGERS: attack, insult, stopped from reaching goal.
   - INDIRECT TRIGGERS: observation, appraisal, thoughts.
2. BECOME AWARE OF AUTOMATIC THOUGHTS associated with anger.
3. CHANGE YOUR THOUGHTS ABOUT THE TRIGGER:
   - CALM DOWN before reacting.
   - THINK ABOUT SITUATION. QUESTION YOUR REACTION.
   - ANOTHER INTERPRETATION?
   - THINK ABOUT NEGATIVE CONSEQUENCES of acting angry.
   - REPLACE NEGATIVE THOUGHTS WITH POSITIVE THOUGHTS.
4. CHANGE WHAT YOU DO:
   - THINK ABOUT OPTIONS.
   - CHOOSE EFFECTIVE BEHAVIOR: makes you calmer or solves problem.
   - AFTERWARDS, LET GO OF THOUGHTS.
   - PLAN ACTIVITY TO COUNTERACT BAD FEELINGS:
     - Call a sober friend to calm down or ask advice about a problem.
     - Do something fun.

Reminder Sheet: Anger Management

Anger often results from the way we think about things:

Trigger Events → Thoughts → Anger → Behavior

- Become more aware of the events and thoughts that trigger your anger.
- Use phrases like these first, to help you calm down in a crisis:

Slow down.	Chill out.
Take it easy.	Easy does it.
Take a deep breath.	Relax.
Cool it.	Count to 10.

- Next, think about what's getting you so angry:
  What's getting me angry? What event? What thoughts?
- Is there another way to interpret the situation?
  Is this really a personal attack or insult?
  Am I overreacting? Is it really that bad?
- Think about the negative consequences of getting angry and the positive consequences of staying cool.
- Replace the negative thoughts with more positive thoughts:
  I don't have to let jerks bother me.
  Life's too short to sweat the small stuff.
  It's not worth risking my sobriety.
- Think about your options:
  What can I do?
  What is in my best interests here?
  Anger should be a signal to start problem solving.
- Do something to make yourself calmer or to solve the problem:
  Leave the situation or take time out.
  Make an assertive request for change.
  Analyze how to deal with the problem.
  Talk to the person in a calm, rational way.
- If the problem won't go away or if you still feel angry:
  Remember that you can't fix everything.
  Try to shake it off. Don't let it interfere with your sobriety.
  Plan something fun to make yourself feel better.
  Call a sober friend to help you calm down.

PRACTICE EXERCISE

Until the next session, pay attention to your response to anger-provoking situations. Try to identify and change your thoughts in those situations. Pick one occasion before the next session involving angry feelings (or feelings of annoyance, frustration, irritation) and record the following:

Trigger situation: _____

_____

_____

_____

(continued)

_____

Reminder Sheet: Anger Management (page 2 of 2)

Calm-down phrases used: _____

_____

_____

_____

Anger-increasing thoughts: _____

_____

_____

_____

Anger-reducing thoughts: _____

_____

_____

_____

Actions to feel calmer or solve the problem: _____

_____

_____

_____

Therapist Tip Sheet: Managing Negative Thinking

POINTS FOR RATIONALE

1. Depression, loneliness, guilt and tension can set the stage for drinking.
   Often results from the way we think about events.
2. Thinking negatively can lead to negative emotions, which can lead to drinking as escape.
3. Negative thinking can become a self-fulfilling prophecy.
   Recognize negative moods as signals to change negative thinking.
   Thoughts can be called "self-talk." Negative thoughts can be AA's "stinking thinking."
4. It takes time and practice before you will notice results.
5. Situations don't make us feel bad; our thoughts about situations result in the feelings. (Give overview, examples of behavior chain.)

POINTS FOR BLACKBOARD (IN CAPITALS)

BEHAVIOR CHAIN

TRIGGER		THOUGHTS/BELIEFS		FEELINGS		BEHAVIOR
EVENT, SITUATION	→	NEGATIVE THOUGHTS	→	FEEL BAD	→	DESTRUCTIVE
		POSITIVE THOUGHTS	→	FEEL GOOD	→	CONSTRUCTIVE

SKILL GUIDELINES

1. MAIN STEPS TO CHANGE:
   - CATCH YOURSELF THINKING NEGATIVELY. Awareness, moods as signal.
   - CHALLENGE AND REPLACE NEGATIVE THOUGHTS.
2. IDENTIFY YOUR NEGATIVE THOUGHTS—generate a list of examples:
   - UNREALISTIC GOALS (perfectionism: should, have to)
   - CATASTROPHIZING (awful, terrible)
   - OVERGENERALIZATION (never, always, no one, everyone)
   - EXPECTING THE WORST
   - SELF-PUT-DOWNS (I don't deserve, I'm no good)
   - BLACK-AND-WHITE THINKING (all or nothing, extremes)
3. CHALLENGE THOUGHTS, REPLACE WITH HEALTHIER THOUGHTS:
   - Challenge premise, realism, interpretation.
   - Replace with moderate, more realistic alternatives.
   - It takes practice to feel effects.
   TYPES OF HEALTHIER THOUGHTS:
   - THINK ABOUT GOOD THINGS ABOUT YOUR LIFE, YOURSELF.
   - CHALLENGE UNREALISTIC OR IRRATIONAL BELIEFS.
   - DECATASTROPHIZE (examine probability, ability to handle).
   - RELABEL DISTRESS (as signal to solve problem).
   - Replace pessimism with HOPEFULNESS STATEMENTS.
   - BLAME EVENT, NOT YOURSELF.
   - STAY ON TASK.
   - REINFORCE YOURSELF (praise self).
4. AFTERWARDS, CHANGE BEHAVIOR: Plan to solve problem.

Reminder Sheet: Managing Negative Thinking

These are the main ways to change negative thinking:

- Events → Thoughts/beliefs → Feelings → Behavior
- Catch negative self-talk whenever you feel upset by an event or crave a drink.
- Identify your negative thoughts:
  - Unrealistic goals or expecting perfection (of self or others): Watch for "should."
  - Catastrophizing: Making a disaster out of an unpleasant event.
  - Overgeneralizing: Watch for "never," "always."
  - Expecting the worst: Watch for "never," "no one," "failure."
  - Self-put-downs: "I don't deserve . . . ," "I'm no good."
  - Black-and-white thinking: all or nothing thoughts.
- Challenge your negative self-talk and replace with positive self-talk.
  - Challenge negativism by remembering the good things about yourself and your life.
  - Challenge irrational beliefs and unrealistic expectations: marked by words like "should," "must," "have to," "awful," "terrible," "disaster," "always," "never," "no one."
  - Decatastrophize: How likely is it and how bad is it really?
  - Relabel distress as a signal to cope
  - Give yourself encouragement and hope.
  - Blame the event or behavior, not the person.
  - Remember to focus on what needs to be done.
  - Give yourself credit for making positive changes.
- Afterwards, change your behavior: Make a plan to solve the problem.

PRACTICE EXERCISE

Use this worksheet to write down one or two events that occur before the next session, your negative thoughts or self-talk, and then your positive thoughts or constructive challenge to the self-talk.

(A) Event or situation	(B) Thoughts/self-talk	
	Negative thoughts →	*Substitute* positive thoughts or *challenge* the negative thoughts
_____	_____	_____
_____	_____	_____
_____	_____	_____
_____	_____	_____
_____	_____	_____
_____	_____	_____

Therapist Tip Sheet: Seemingly Irrelevant Decisions

POINTS FOR RATIONALE WITH POINTS FOR BLACKBOARD (IN CAPITALS)

1. Little decisions, seemingly ordinary, can move you closer to relapse.
2. Need to learn ways you may SET YOURSELF UP FOR RELAPSE THROUGH MINOR DECISIONS that seem to have nothing to do with drinking.
3. THINK AHEAD ABOUT EVERY CHOICE you make, WHERE EACH MAY LEAD, ANTICIPATE DANGERS.
4. CHOOSE LOW-RISK OPTIONS to avoid potentially risky situations.
5. IF YOU CHOOSE RISKY OPTION, PLAN HOW TO PROTECT YOURSELF in high-risk situation.
6. Example: Stu left half hour early, detoured through downtown (supposedly to watch construction), parked by familiar bar, got change for meter in the bar, saw old friend in bar and stayed to talk with him, friend bought Stu a beer without asking, Stu thought it would be rude to refuse, relapsed.
7. AWARENESS INCREASES ABILITY to take corrective actions, avoid high-risk situations. Easier to handle high-risk situations before you get too close than in the middle.

GROUP DISCUSSION

Discuss following examples:
- Keeping liquor in house for guests.
- Going to bar to see friends, sports on TV, eat, play darts, use phone.
- Going to party where people are drinking.
- Keeping secret from your friends that you quit drinking.
- Where to go for snack (e.g., liquor store or gas station).
- Route to drive (e.g. passing a favorite bar or liquor store vs. detour).
- Taking a job as bartender or in liquor store.
- Not making plans for weekend.
- Telling a friend that you have quit drinking.
- Planning how to spend free time after work.
- Starting conversation with people at AA or NA meetings.
- Asking housemate not to bring alcohol into the house.

Reminder Sheet: Seemingly Irrelevant Decisions

Little decisions that each seem ordinary can move you closer to relapse. When making any decision, whether large or small, do the following:

- Consider what options you may have.
- Think ahead to the possible outcomes of each option. What positive or negative consequences can you anticipate, and what are the risks of relapse?
- Select one of the options:
  Choose one that will minimize your relapse risk.
  If you decide to choose a risky option, plan how to protect yourself while in the high-risk situation.

PRACTICE EXERCISE

Think about a decision you have made recently or are about to make. The decision could involve any aspect of your life, such as your job, recreational activities, friends, or family. Identify "safe" choices and choices that might increase your odds of relapsing.

Decision to be made: _____

_____

_____

_____

_____

_____

Safe alternatives: _____

_____

_____

_____

_____

_____

Risky alternatives: _____

_____

_____

_____

_____

_____

Therapist Tip Sheet: Planning for Emergencies

POINTS FOR RATIONALE

1. Important to plan in advance how to handle crises.
2. Some disruptive life events or changes can led to relapse.
   - Separations (e.g., divorce, death, child leaving, friends moving away)
   - Health problems
   - New responsibilities (e.g., promotion, new child, volunteering)
   - Adjustment to new situations
   - Work-related events (e.g., job loss, new job, promotion)
   - Financial changes
3. Positive events can also pose a risk (e.g., marriage, moving, promotion, graduation):
   - Involve many changes in lifestyle.
   - New responsibilities can increase stress.
   - Feeling like celebrating can lead to relapse.
   - Overconfidence.
4. Major events of family or friends can affect you, increase risk of relapse.

POINTS FOR BLACKBOARD (IN CAPITALS)

LIST LIFE EVENTS OR CHANGES you can anticipate
Get examples from group.

SKILL GUIDELINES

1. WHAT SKILLS CAN BE USED IN YOUR PLAN?
   Problem solving
   Monitoring decisions
   Managing thoughts about drinking, anger, or negative thoughts
   Increasing pleasant events
2. PREPARE A GENERAL EMERGENCY PLAN:
   Problem-solving skills
   Calling people for support
   Increase going to AA or NA
   Challenging, replacing negative thoughts
   Increasing pleasant activities
   What else?

Reminder Sheet: Planning for Emergencies

Plan ahead for coping with possible unexpected stressful events.

- Think about problem-solving skills: What can you do to handle the problem?
- Consider who you can call for support.
- Increase going to AA or NA.
- Think about how to manage your emotions (e.g., anger, urges, depression).
- Think about pleasant activities that could counteract your negative feelings.

PRACTICE EXERCISE

Write a detailed emergency plan for coping with situations that could pose a high risk for relapse. Be specific about each possible coping strategy (e.g., which meeting you would you go to, where, and how you would get there?).

1. _____
_____
_____
_____

2. _____
_____
_____
_____

3. _____
_____
_____
_____

4. _____
_____
_____
_____

5. _____
_____
_____
_____

FIVE

Cue Exposure Treatment
with Urge Coping Training

Conceptual Overview   132
Methodological Issues   133
Assessments   138
Conducting CET with Urge-Specific Coping Skills Training   140
Individual Differences in Cue Reactivity   148
Copies of Measures   151
Therapist Tip Sheets   155
Reminder Sheet   162

CONCEPTUAL OVERVIEW

During and after treatment, alcoholics encounter a variety of alcohol-related cues in the environment. By cues we mean people, places, objects, time periods, and internal states that have been associated with drinking in the past. Cues can include the sight and smell of one's favorite alcoholic beverage; places such as bars, beaches, and homes where drinking occurred; mood states such as stress, anger, or wanting to celebrate; certain times, such as the end of work or Friday evening; and people who had been drinking companions. Because alcoholics are asked to avoid drinking cues while in treatment, our clients may first encounter these cues outside of the treatment setting unexpectedly, and with no one present to help them deal with their internal reactions to the cues, posing a risk for relapse. Cue exposure treatment (CET) was developed to help clients reduce the strength of the internal reactions and to practice using coping skills while in the state of arousal that these cues generate.

CET is derived from classical learning theory and social learning theory models of the relationship between alcohol-related cues and relapse (described further in Monti & Rohsenow, 1999). These models propose that both environmental and internal cues associated with drinking in the past can produce conditioned reactions (such as when a dog salivates to the sound of the can opener working), and that these reactions may play a role in triggering a relapse to drinking (Niaura et al., 1988; Rohsenow, Monti, & Abrams, 1995). These reactions can interfere with an alcoholic's attempts to cope in a high-risk situation. Therefore, the chance to practice using coping skills while experiencing the internal reactions that result from the presence of alcohol cues can increase the likelihood that the client will be able to use these skills effectively when later encountering cues. It may also be that much drinking behavior is controlled by automatic, overlearned cognitive networks; like any habitual behavior, drinking occurs without much conscious thought (Tiffany, 1990). In the presence of alcohol cues, the conditioned reactions may set the stage for automatic alcohol-seeking behavior to occur without much awareness. Teaching alcoholics to focus attention on these reactions and on urge to drink in the presence of cues may increase their awareness of danger and increase the likelihood of mobilizing coping skills to keep from drinking (Rohsenow et al., 1994; Monti, Rohsenow, & Hutchison, 2000).

CET can have several kinds of effects. First, repeated exposure to a cue while preventing the drinking response should result in habituation (i.e., decrease in strength) of the conditioned reactions over time. However, habituation tends to occur to the specific cues used, and the reaction is easily reinstated if the alcoholic sees a different cue, so a wide variety of cues are needed in treatment. Second, practice in using coping skills in the presence of alcohol cues should make it easier to use these skills effectively in the presence of cues, and increase alcoholics' beliefs that they can respond effectively to cues. In these ways, internal reactions to alcohol cues should interfere less with the alcoholic's ability to use his/her skills in the real world after treatment. Therefore, we combine exposure with coping skills practice to allow both processes to occur.

METHODOLOGICAL ISSUES IN CONDUCTING CUE EXPOSURE

In this section, we discuss some of the methodological issues to consider when designing the CET approach. These clinical issues involve different ways in which the CET could be done, based on what is known to date, and indicate the size of the task that confronts future clinicians and researchers.

Safety Issues and Setting

Because CET produces elevated urges to drink and other reactions that do not necessarily dissipate completely by the end of the session, the setting in which it is conducted needs to be thoughtfully considered, to provide the best protection for the clients. The optimal setting is an inpatient or residential one, so that any residual effects of the exposure sessions can be handled by clinical staff, without any danger that the client will leave and drink. However, with managed care, this may not be possible. The next preferred, less restrictive setting is a day treatment program, in which clients are on site for 4–8 hours per day, and CET is conducted earlier in the day, so that 2 or more hours of additional treatment time follow in which residual reactions can be handled. A benefit of this outpatient setting is opportunities for between-session practice of urge coping skills as naturally occurring exposure opportunities arise. It is even possible to assign exposure homework to clients (e.g., Blakey & Baker, 1980), but it is more difficult to ensure that drinking does not occur during exposure without the therapist's presence. Least safe is for CET to occur in outpatient sessions that are not embedded in a day treatment or partial hospital program. If the client leaves immediately after the CET session, it is more difficult to ensure that residual reactions will not lead to drinking. If outpatient treatment is to be conducted, the client should have a clear commitment to the treatment goal, adherence to the treatment goal should be assessed at the start of every session, and CET should be replaced with another form of treatment if the client has not adhered to the goal. We have conducted CET or laboratory alcohol-exposure sessions with many hundreds of alcohol-dependent clients without a single relapse being attributed to the exposure. Therefore, with treatment-motivated clients and sufficient safeguards, it is possible to conduct CET safely.

A related issue is that CET is not designed to be the sole treatment that alcoholics receive. Alcohol dependence is a complex issue and needs a comprehensive approach to treatment. If contributing issues such as vocational, psychiatric, medical, social, and family needs are not addressed, these issues may precipitate relapse. CET is designed to be a useful adjunct to a comprehensive alcohol treatment program by addressing an aspect of recovery not usually covered.

Additional safety precautions should be taken. Clients are never left alone with beverages, and we ensure that no other clients ever see or smell the beverages or empty containers. Furthermore, clients are instructed that avoidance remains the best strategy, and that exposure should never be done on one's own.

Relevant Cues for Exposure

The types of stimuli that a therapist could use for cue exposure can vary widely, particularly because such a wide variety of cues typically have become associated with drinking for any one client. The task is to narrow down the field to the most relevant cues.

Beverage Cues

The client's favorite alcohol beverage is one obvious choice, because the sight and smell of the beverage is the final common pathway in the chain of behaviors leading to drinking. One study showed that the more similar the drink was to the alcoholic's customary beverage, the stronger he/she reacted in terms of desire to drink, withdrawal symptoms, and heart rate (Staiger & White, 1991). Furthermore, the sight and smell of the favorite drink produced stronger reactions than did the sight alone of the same drink, indicating that every client should be asked to smell the drink as well as look at it.

Other Triggers

Another issue is whether the beverage exposure alone is sufficient, because it is the common final pathway before drinking, or whether other types of cues should be included. Learning theory suggests that it is easier to stop a chain of responses when intervening further away from the final behavior (drinking) than when close to the final step (i.e., when the drink is in hand), indicating that exposure trials should occur with more distal triggers as well. Also, about one-third to one-half of the alcoholics we have studied failed to react to the presence of their preferred beverage (Cooney, Litt, Gaupp, & Schmidt, 1989; Rohsenow et al., 1992). Alcoholics who do not react to the beverage usually can identify situations or events that will elicit a strong urge to drink. The chain of behaviors that lead to drinking commonly includes many elements before beverage stimuli appear, including other people, events, thoughts, and emotional states, and these other elements may trigger the motivation to seek alcohol. Although these complex stimuli can be hard to present for real in the treatment setting, especially triggers such as an argument or a phone call from one's ex, these triggers can be experienced by clients by using imaginal techniques.

Mood induction is another method of producing imaginal exposure, by using guided imagery to generate mood states that have commonly preceded drinking for the individual client (Cooney, Litt, Morse, Bauer, & Gaupp, 1997; Litt, Cooney, Kadden, & Gaupp, 1990; Rubonis et al., 1994). Embedding the targeted mood state within the context of the particular situation that commonly evoked a drinking episode should create a particularly powerful combination of conditioned stimuli. The mood induction procedure may be particularly relevant for women: in one study, urge to drink was increased after a negative mood induction based on a high-risk drinking situation for women but not for men (Rubonis et al., 1994).

Alcohol Ingestion as a Cue for Heavy Drinking

A controversial issue derived from the theoretical models is whether limited alcohol ingestion should be included in CET. In most U.S. treatment facilities, alcohol ingestion is not an option, but in some other countries, such as Great Britain, limited alcohol ingestion has been included as a cue (e.g., Rankin, Hodgson, & Stockwell, 1983). This choice is used only in programs with a treatment goal of moderate drinking, so that excessive drinking is the response being eliminated, rather than all drinking. The choice is based on conceptualizing the conditioned stimulus to be limited alcohol ingestion and its effects, with continued drinking being the emitted response that is targeted for prevention. However, treatment goal issues aside, this may not be the best point in the behavior chain at which to intervene. Because it is harder for people to interrupt a chain of behaviors close to the final behavior (Bandura, 1977), greater effectiveness is likely if clients are helped to interrupt the behavior chain before drinking.

Individualized versus Standardized Sets of Cues

Another methodological issue is whether cues should be individually tailored to specific clients or whether all clients can receive the same set of standardized drinking cues in CET. Some studies using CET with opiate, cocaine, and alcohol abusers have used standardized stimuli (Dawe & Powell, 1995; Drummond & Glautier, 1994; Rankin et al., 1983), whereas other studies with alcoholics have employed individually tailored sets of stimuli based on analyses of the clients' drinking (Blakey & Baker, 1980; Hodgson & Rankin, 1982; Monti, Rohsenow, Rubonis, Niaura, Sirota, Colby, Goddard, & Abrams, 1993). Based on learning theories and the variety of high-risk situations that clients report, individualized cues should be the preferred method.

Order of Presentation of Cues

Exposure-based treatments usually present stimuli in a hierarchy, but the order of the hierarchy is debatable. CET was derived essentially from exposure-based treatment for anxiety, which found that the order in which conditioned stimuli are presented is irrelevant to treatment success (e.g., Leitenberg, 1976). Hodgson (1989) recommended that stimuli be presented in a graduated order, starting with the less tempting stimuli before presenting more urge-provoking stimuli. However, in this era of managed care, we prefer to start with the most urge-provoking stimuli (Monti, Rohsenow, Rubonis, Niaura, Sirota, Colby, Goddard, & Abrams, 1993; Monti, Rohsenow, Colby, & Abrams, 1995). We begin each session with the sight and smell of the client's customary alcoholic beverage; then, with the beverage in sight, we ask clients to imagine being in various high-risk situations, starting with the situation they think would cause the greatest urge to drink. This is tolerated well by alcoholic clients.

Individual versus Group-Administered CET

Individual CET sessions make it easier to manage individualized sets of stimuli. Individual sessions also have the advantage of allowing the length of exposure time to be based on the individual client's response, and make it easier to explore thoughts the client has when urges go up and when they later decrease during exposure. However, group sessions of exposure are also possible. In one study (Monti et al., 2001), groups of three to five clients were provided CET by standardizing the length of time each client was exposed to the beverage and imaginal triggers. For each exposure, 8 minutes was allowed (3 minutes for the urge to rise, and 5 minutes for them to practice using the urge-specific coping skill), and the beverage and imaginal triggers were each individualized. A second study conducted CET in groups of three or four clients in which a priming dose of alcohol was consumed followed by simply looking at an additional drink for two 9-minute trials per session (Sitharthan, Sitharthan, Hough, & Kavanaugh, 1997). While individual exposure is preferable, group exposure is possible if the constraints of the setting do not permit individual treatment.

Attention Focus during Exposure

Alcoholics often try to avoid focusing on the drinking-related stimuli, or on their responses to the stimuli, because of the aversiveness of the temptation to drink. The avoidance may be visual (looking elsewhere) or cognitive (distraction). However, failure to attend may decrease the effectiveness of cue exposure, because habituation may not occur if the conditioned responses are not elicited. In studies of CET with patients with anxiety disorders, attention-focusing instructions were found to produce greater habituation between sessions than instructions for patients to distract themselves from the stimuli (Grayson, Foa, & Steketee, 1982; Sartory, Rachman, & Grey, 1982). Also, alcoholics in a lab study, who reported that they had paid more attention to either the beverage stimuli or to their physiological reactions to those stimuli, drank less often during the next 3 months (Rohsenow et al., 1994). For these reasons, we recommend that clients be instructed to focus on both the stimuli and on their reactions to the stimuli during CET.

Nature of the Response Being Monitored for Change

When drinking triggers are organized into hierarchies, this is usually done on the basis of relative degree of urge or desire to drink expected in the situation (e.g., Monti, Rohsenow, Rubonis, Niaura, Sirota, Colby, Goddard, & Abrams, 1993; Rankin et al., 1983). In the treatment sessions, urge or desire to drink during exposure is usually monitored through self-report, in addition to ensuring that the behavioral response (e.g., holding the beverage) is carried out. While cue-elicited salivation has been shown to be a better predictor of posttreatment drinking than has cue-elicited urge to drink (see Monti, Rohsenow, & Hutchison, 2000), salivation would be too difficult to measure on an ongoing basis throughout CET sessions. Skin conductance is the one other psychophysiological response that has been reliably elicited by cues (Rohsenow et al., 1990). Although it is difficult to monitor skin conductance throughout treatment sessions due to movement artifacts, this was successfully done in one treatment trial and was found to predict treatment outcome (Drummond & Glautier, 1994). However, for most clinical purposes, urge, desire, or temptation to drink are more feasible to monitor, as well as having face validity. The key element is that exposure occurs during the sessions. As long as exposure is occurring, the whole network of conditioned responses is presumed to have a chance to habituate.

Dosage and Regimen

Sessions should be long enough for within-session habituation to stimuli to occur. Studies of CET with anxiety-based disorders have found that longer sessions (50–90 minutes) are more beneficial than shorter ones, and exposure four or more times per week works better than less frequent exposure (Foa & Kozak, 1986; Marks, 1987). With opiate abusers as well, 45 minutes to 1 hour of exposure is more effective than 10 minutes of exposure per session (see Dawe & Powell, 1995; Childress, McLellan, & O'Brien, 1985; Rankin et al., 1983).

Some alcohol literature suggests guidelines for the length and timing of CET sessions. In a laboratory study, alcoholics were exposed to the sight and smell of their preferred beverage for 18 minutes, followed by another 15 minutes of exposure to the sight alone. In this study, urge peaked at 6 minutes, decreased significantly over the next 12 minutes of sight and smell combined, and continued a smooth significant descent over the subsequent 15 minutes of visual exposure (Monti, Rohsenow, Rubonis, Niaura, Sirota, Colby, & Abrams, 1993). Another similar study that used 20-minute exposure to the sight and smell of the preferred beverage found significant decreases in desire to drink, withdrawal symptoms, and heart rate (Staiger & White, 1991). In that study, self-report measures stabilized within 13 minutes, and effects on heart rate stabilized within 9 minutes. These studies suggested that significant within-session habituation can occur relatively rapidly, within 18–20 minutes of exposure, and can continue to occur when only visual exposure is continued.

Some guidance is available from controlled treatment trials for the number of trials needed for CET with alcoholics. Significant decreases in cue reactivity and improvement in drinking outcomes were obtained with six 55-minute sessions of CET in one study (Monti, Rohsenow, Rubonis, Niaura, Sirota, Colby, Goddard, & Abrams, 1993) and with 7.5–8 50-minute sessions in another study (Rohsenow et al., 2001). Significant treatment results were found with ten 40-minute trials by Drummond and Glautier (1994) and with six 90-

minute sessions by Sitharthan et al. (1997). Based on the combined literature regarding alcohol and opiate abusers, we currently recommend at least six or seven sessions that are 45–60 minutes in length for effective CET.

Passive Exposure versus Active Coping during CET

In the classical learning models, exposure alone should result in habituation or extinction of the conditioned response, and be sufficient for effective treatment. However, generalization might not occur from cues used in the treatment sessions to cues in the environment, as was shown with opiate abusers (Childress, McLellan, Ehrman, & O'Brien, 1988), and simple exposure may be aversive and lead to early termination. Furthermore, it may be beneficial to teach coping methods in the context of alcohol-related cues, as described earlier. Therefore, the CET approaches of several groups of researchers include teaching and practicing skills for coping with urges to drink or use drugs (Childress, 1993; Cooney et al., 1993; Monti, Rohsenow, Rubonis, Niaura, Sirota, Colby, Goddard, & Abrams, 1993; Rohsenow et al., 2001). It is important that exposure continue throughout the session while conducting the coping skills training, both for habituation to continue and for skills practice while in the altered state produced by the presence of cues to occur.

ASSESSMENTS

Drinking Triggers Interview

The Drinking Triggers Interview (DTI; Monti, Rohsenow, Rubonis, Niaura, Sirota, Colby, Goddard, & Abrams, 1993; see Form 5.1 at the end of the chapter) is used as the basis for the imaginal exposure to individualized drinking cues. During the imaginal exposure, it is important to expose clients to the most salient triggers of their drinking. By triggers, we mean the people, situations, environments, events, or emotional experiences that often lead to a drinking episode or a strong urge to drink.

The DTI, a structured interview, is easily administered in the office. First, we ask the clients to describe all the situations or events that have been associated with frequent heavy drinking, relapse, or strong urges to drink in the past. We write down the essential elements of each situation. Next, we ask clients to make confidence ratings: "If you were out of the hospital and in this situation today, how confident are you that you could handle this situation without drinking, on a 0–10 scale?" The client is shown a card with the 11 numbers, ranging from "Not at all confident" to "Completely confident." We ask the clients also to rate each situation for urge to drink: "If you were out of the hospital and in this situation today, how strong would your urge to drink be, on a 0–10 scale?" On the card showing this scale, 0 is labeled "No urge at all" and 10 is labeled "Extremely strong urge to drink." Last, we ask the clients to rank-order the situations for the frequency with which they occur. We then order the triggers into a hierarchy based on the strength of the anticipated urge to drink in the situation, with ties broken by ranking the more frequent trigger higher than a less frequently occurring trigger.

> *Note*: Trauma-related triggers are not used as imaginal cues, out of concern that posttraumatic stress may provide too strong a trigger to be handled using cue exposure. Therefore, always screen for trauma-related triggers. Events we avoid using during exposure include the death of a child, rape, any recent deaths, or combat stress. Ask if the trauma memories trigger alcohol use, how often clients think about the event, and whether it would be difficult for them if the trauma event was described during treatment. Events that are infrequently thought of or mild in effect are all right, but events associated with a posttraumatic distress syndrome should not be used except by therapists experienced in conducting exposure therapy for PTSD.

Assessing Urge-Specific Cognitive and Behavioral Coping Skills

The Urge-Specific Strategies Questionnaire (USSQ; see Form 5.2 at the end of the chapter) has been developed as a means of assessing through self-report the coping skills clients use when confronted with urges to drink (Monti, Rohsenow, Rubonis, Niaura, Sirota, Colby, Goddard, & Abrams, 1993; Rohsenow et al., 2001). This can be given before treatment, to determine areas of strengths or weaknesses on which to focus, or after, treatment to assess acquisition of skills.

First, we use an open-ended assessment of clients' coping skills, to find out what they will volunteer without prompting. We ask clients to describe every strategy they have tried when they have had an urge to drink, in order to keep themselves from drinking. These strategies are coded into the types of strategies described below. Then, we provide a list of key coping strategies, worded in plain language. The clients are asked to rate how often they used each strategy when they had an urge to drink and were trying to keep from drinking. The frequency ratings are made on a scale from "Never" (0) to "Every time" (10).

The strategies assessed are the following:

1. Delay.
2. Thinking of negative consequences of drinking.
3. Thinking of positive consequences of sobriety.
4. Alternative food or drink.
5. Alternative behaviors.
6. Meditation or formal relaxation methods.
7. Escape or avoidance.
8. Self-punishment.
9. Willpower alone.

The first five items are strategies we currently recommend teaching in CET; the next two are other strategies commonly taught in treatment programs, and the last two are strategies that are generally found ineffective, as reviewed in our research chapter. In our own research, the strategies that were significantly correlated with reductions in quantity and/ or frequency of drinking during the year following treatment included delay, thinking about positive or negative consequences, alternative consumption or behaviors, and escape or avoidance (Monti et al., 1990; Rohsenow et al., 2001). Other strategies were not positively associated with improvements in drinking behavior.

CONDUCTING CET WITH URGE-SPECIFIC COPING SKILLS TRAINING

Overview of CET

CET has the following basic goals:

1. The client acquires greater knowledge about his/her own set of personal drinking triggers.
2. The client is exposed to these triggers until his/her urge to drink decreases to a low level. This is designed to allow habituation or desensitization to occur.
3. The client learns a set of urge-specific cognitive and behavioral strategies for coping with urges to drink.
4. The client practices these strategies while experiencing real urges to drink, and experiences the effects of these strategies on his/her own urge level.
5. The client learns which strategy is most effective with each specific trigger, and which strategies are not so effective. A strategy that works well with one trigger may not work well with another.
6. The client leaves with a written personalized "toolbox" that lists the strategies as personalized for the particular client, for later review (see Figure 5.2 on p. 144 and Reminder Sheet on p. 162).

Each session starts with a period of intensive exposure to the alcoholic beverage, with the client holding, smelling, and focusing attention on the beverage. Then, we leave the beverage in plain view throughout rest of session so that passive exposure to the beverage continues. Next, we conduct imaginal exposure to other triggers by asking the client to vividly imagine being in trigger situations identified using the DTI. Clients sometimes intensify the exposure experience by handling and looking at the beverage during the imaginal exposure. After each session's first exposure to the beverage and one imaginal scene, we teach a new urge-specific coping skill. Finally, we have the client practice the new skill while engaging in additional periods of imaginal exposure. When the session ends, we put away the beverage in a covered carrier and discuss the client's reactions. The therapist should work to defuse any urge or affect before releasing the client (changing the subject to a distracting topic usually works well).

Introduction and Rationale Presented to Client

Before conducting any CET with the clients, it is necessary to present a rationale and some ground rules to them. We include the following elements in the introduction we give:

"We have found that many people have trouble after treatment because they react
   to triggers that were associated with drinking in the past. While in the treatment

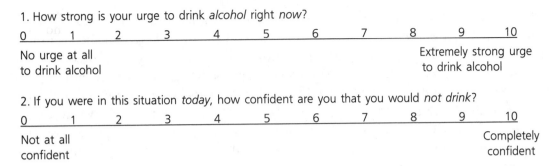

1. How strong is your urge to drink *alcohol* right *now*?

| 0 | 1 | 2 | 3 | 4 | 5 | 6 | 7 | 8 | 9 | 10 |

No urge at all   Extremely strong urge
to drink alcohol   to drink alcohol

2. If you were in this situation *today*, how confident are you that you would *not drink*?

| 0 | 1 | 2 | 3 | 4 | 5 | 6 | 7 | 8 | 9 | 10 |

Not at all   Completely
confident   confident

FIGURE 5.1. Urge and confidence ratings used in treatment.

program, many people stop having cravings because they are away from their drinking triggers. But after leaving the program and first seeing your triggers again, you may have a strong urge to drink, with no one there to help you through it. The best way to deal with drinking triggers is to avoid them completely. However, no one can avoid all drinking triggers: You see beer when watching games on TV or walking down the street, and emotional triggers such as fights or depression can't be avoided. This program is designed to help you learn to resist temptation more easily while in the safety of the treatment program. This is done in two ways: First, we ask you to experience your drinking triggers until you feel the urge to drink decreasing. In this way, you learn that your urges will go away without drinking. Also, you will become more aware of responses you experience, both physical and emotional, to triggers. Second, you will learn ways to make it easier to handle urges. We will teach you some skills and review the skills you already know. Practicing these skills while having urges will make you quicker and more effective in using them later on, when you run into triggers on your own. However, do not practice exposing yourself to drinking triggers on your own. If you test yourself and fail, you will have wasted this treatment. The goal is not to make you able to deliberately expose yourself to triggers, but rather to help you deal better with triggers that you can't avoid."

We define what we mean by urge: "By an urge, we mean how much you want, wish, crave, or thirst for alcohol." We put on the table a card on which is printed the first urge rating scale from Figure 5.1 and explain how to use the 0–10 rating scale. We add that when clients report their urge to us using numbers, it is like a thermometer, allowing us to know what is going on inside of them. Clients all respond well to this approach to reporting their level of urge.

Beverage Exposure

Each session begins with beverage exposure. We do this because the beverage is always the final stimulus that alcoholics are exposed to in real life, before they drink, so we want to desensitize this final common pathway to drinking. It is important to use the client's customary alcoholic beverage(s), prepared in his/her usual way. If the person drinks Popov red label vodka with Pepsi on the rocks in a tall glass, this is what is presented, along with the commercially labeled bottles for the two beverages. Timing the length of the exposure is useful for giving the client feedback about how much more quickly the urge decreases across sessions. If you do this, start a stopwatch when you bring the beverage into view. Ask the client to pour and mix the drink (without filling the glass) while reporting every change in urge to drink using the 0–10 scale. Then ask if his/her urge is greater when holding, looking at, or sniffing the glass or the bottle/can. "Focus on whatever aspect of the drink gives a greater urge—the sight, smell, feel of the glass, thoughts. Try to experience the greatest urge you can." Many clients have less urge when smelling the drink than when looking at it. If asked, most clients report that when drinking, they never take their hand off of the bottle/can/glass, so ask them to do likewise during CET. Watch for attempts to avoid looking at the beverage or to lean away; encourage clients to focus on it.

When the urge is as high as the client thinks it will go, the delay procedure or coping skill practice is implemented, as described below. After this is completed, ask the client what he/she was thinking about, and discuss aspects of the stimuli that brought the urge up, and what he/she was thinking when the urge came down. It is important to know what clients were actually thinking about during the exposure rather than to assume that they were thinking what they were instructed to think. This provides knowledge of their barriers and spontaneous use of coping. Time from peak to lowest urge is shown to clients in later sessions to show them their progress in reducing urges more quickly, and to identify the most effective coping strategies for them.

Sometimes clients do not report urges in response to the beverage, and this needs to be discussed. First, not everyone has an urge in response to alcohol cues. Instead, many are affected only by emotional or situational cues. With these people, conduct exposure for 8 minutes each session anyway, because autonomic reactions may be occurring that can be habituated through exposure. Second, some clients do not let themselves respond. Deal with resistance by letting them know that this treatment can only work if they let themselves experience the urge. Remind them that this is a safe place, and tell them that the urge will mostly go away after the session is over. Third, some clients avoid looking at or touching the glass and need to be redirected. Let clients know this approach only works well if they let themselves feel the urge, and that suppressing urges might result in a rebound effect later on. Although we do not know that it is necessary to feel the urge, we try to prevent cognitive avoidance in sessions, so that clients can practice handling urges in this safe environment and experience the results.

Conducting Imaginal Scene Exposure

The DTI is the primary source of scenes for the imaginal exposure, but any new situations that come up during the CET can be added to the list and used during exposure. We always start with the highest ranked trigger (highest urge rating with ties broken by frequency) for two reasons. First, we want people to have as much practice as possible with their most difficult triggers. Therefore, we start every session with the same imaginal trigger—the one reported to be the strongest one originally. Second, people gain confidence as they see the rapidity with which urges in their most feared triggers decrease over sessions. Across sessions, there are two different considerations to keep in mind when selecting triggers for exposure:

1. Be sure to include all the triggers across sessions to maximize generalization.
2. Be sure to conduct repeated exposures to the stronger triggers, to maximize habituation of responses.

Before presenting each trigger scene, ask the client to provide more details about aspects of the situation that increase his/her urge to drink. Then, ask the client to vividly imagine being in the situation and to focus on the elements that lead to the greatest urge to drink. It is important to ask the client to imagine being in the situation after he/she leaves treatment and to imagine that he/she still plans to stay sober. The client should not imagine the past, when he/she was planning to drink. The client is told not to imagine drinking in the situation or escaping from it. Having clients imagine the scene themselves is usually more effective than trying to narrate it for them. Ask them to report their urge every time it changes. Then if their urge fails to increase, or fails to decrease after coping skills are applied, stop them, ask them to describe exactly what they were thinking about, and give corrective feedback. For example, one client was imagining drinking and another kept changing the situation by adding new stimulus elements to prevent habituation.

Ask clients to focus on imagining the elements that lead to the greatest urge. It usually takes between 1 second and 2 minutes for the urge to reach its maximum. When their urge is as high as they think it will go, engage in the delay procedure or coping skills practice described below. Once again, after the scene is terminated, ask for details about their thoughts while imagining the scene, and when applying the skills, so as to troubleshoot problems and learn about uninstructed stimuli or skills they are including. The same methods of handling resistance described earlier are applied to the imaginal scenes.

Practicing Urge Coping Skills during Exposure

The first beverage exposure and the first imaginal exposure are conducted using the delay procedure (below) in the first session and practicing the coping skill taught in the previous session in later sessions. After these first two exposures are terminated, teach a new coping skill. When teaching, first describe the coping method and personalize it by having clients generate examples of the method that they think would work for them. Write these personal examples down in a written Personal Toolbox that you can use as suggestions during CET, and that the client will keep at the end of treatment (see Figure 5.2 and Reminder Sheet at the end of the chapter). Then, have the client again engage in imaginal exposure or beverage exposure, and when the urge is elevated, have him/her imagine using the coping skill while in the situation.

For situations such as an argument with someone, the coping strategy cannot be applied in the midst of it, because the client is too busy interacting. The greatest danger is just afterwards, when the client would normally leave and go get a drink or drive to a liquor store. In such cases, have the client imagine having the fight, then hanging up the phone and sitting down, or leaving the house and sitting in the car without driving, before practicing the coping strategy. If the client keeps moving in the scene, we have found that he/she will go get a drink, so the client needs to learn to stop and think through the coping while in a safe place.

The coping practice is conducted as follows: When the urge is as high as the client thinks it will go, ask him/her to practice one of the coping strategies while imagining he/she is still in the scene. For example, "Stay in the scene, vividly imagining it, but now think about all the good things that would happen if you stayed sober. You are still there, but you are thinking about the good things that would happen to your family and your finances if

1. **Things I can say to help me wait it out:**
   - Tell myself that the urge will go down with time.
   - I can wait it out.

2. **Negative results if I started to drink again:**
   - Marriage in great jeopardy.
   - Impair ability to paint and do other hobbies.
   - Any future employment would be gone.
   - Family would feel disgust and disappointment; they'd watch me. Father would change will.
   - Having to go into a hospital/rehab again.
   - Having to go through withdrawal and detox again.
   - Having to face the people in detox.
   - If I live long, quality of life will be zero for a long time.

3. **Positive results of sobriety for me:**
   - More creative: can paint, write a novel.
   - Marriage better: do more activities together, have more freedom in what we do together, more peace and pleasure.
   - Health: would feel better, have more energy.
   - Financial situation will be better, because I'll be able to work.
   - Self-esteem, self-confident, do things very well.
   - Have respect from children and friends.
   - Spiritually energized and attuned.
   - Would be able to keep living in the house.

4. **Eat or drink something else:**
   - Drink a mocha (coffee + hot chocolate)
   - Eat a dish of ice cream.
   - As distracting thing to do or as a reward for resisting urge.

5. **Do something else:**
   - Pray.
   - Walk.
   - Drive to the shore.
   - Paint.
   - Read an escape novel.
   - Watch TV or videotape.

FIGURE 5.2. Example: Joe's Personal Toolbox for reducing urges.

you stayed sober." Terminate the scene when the urge is as low as you think it will go but at least a 2 or lower on the scale. Usually, it takes between 15 seconds and 10 minutes for the urge to decrease to its minimum. In the first session, there may only be time for one or two imaginal exposures in total, but over time, more exposure periods can be conducted in each CET session.

After terminating the exposure, ask clients what they were thinking about when first imagining the scene, and after applying the skill. Help them notice which coping skills work best with which scenes. In later sessions, have them practice not only the new skill taught the previous session but also other, previous skills. One goal is to have them try a variety of the coping strategies with each of the imaginal scenes, to help them identify which skills work best in which situations. We generally find that thinking about negative consequences works better for positive- than negative-affect situations, possibly because compounding the negative affect through negative consequences makes the trigger stronger. Similarly, thinking about negative consequences may be more effective than thinking about positive ones in positive social situations. Alternative food or drink is likely to be more effective when at home watching TV, or at a party, than when having a fight with someone. Clients can write this information in their Personal Toolbox.

In the early sessions, we tell the clients which tools to use with each trigger to ensure sufficient practice of each strategy. In the first beverage and imaginal exposure of the session, have them use the strategy taught in the previous session. Then, teach a new tool and have clients practice that tool with imaginal exposure. Next, match each strategy to each different trigger, so that they experience which strategies work better or worse with each trigger. During the last two sessions, instead of always telling clients which coping strategy to practice, at times, ask them to use any method, or combination of methods, to get the urge down. This encourages generalization by having clients practice free recall of the coping and combining strategies. For example, after a fight with a family member, in addition to reminding him/herself of the consequences of drinking, the client may want to plan an alternative activity that would lift his/her mood (go get a pizza) or provide social support (call a best buddy).

At the end of each session, ask clients to practice using these skills whenever they experience an urge between sessions. Anticipate any situations that might result in an urge before the next session, especially in a session before the weekend, and have clients discuss the coping strategies they want to use. However, remind them not to deliberately expose themselves to cues. At the start of each session, ask whether any urges occurred, and how it went when they tried coping with the urges. This practice aids generalization. During the last session, review all the strategies used, summarize which ones worked best in which situations, and remind clients of the importance of practicing these new skills. We like to type up clients' Personal Toolboxes and provide them with a printed copy for easy reference. (See Reminder Sheet at the end of the chapter.)

Urge-Specific Coping Strategies

The following urge-specific coping strategies were chosen based on previous literature as most likely to be effective in urge coping and to be applicable immediately after experiencing an urge. The only strategies we ask clients not to rehearse mentally are the following:

1. Escape or avoidance, because we want to maximize exposure to allow desensitization or habituation to occur. We do tell them that escape and avoidance are the best strategies to use, but that in these sessions we want them to practice only other methods.
2. Self-punishment, because work with smokers has shown that it increases the likelihood of relapse (Shiffman, 1984).
3. Willpower alone, because research with smokers has shown that it is half as effective as any other strategy (Shiffman, 1984). Although clients may say that willpower or escape and avoidance are all they need, we point out that it is useful to have as many tools in their toolbox as possible, in case they get into a situation that is harder to handle.

We ask clients to try out all these tools and see for themselves which ones work best. We have also taught urge-reduction imagery (Marlatt & Gordon, 1985), mastery statements, and cognitive distraction. However, those strategies were not correlated with drinking outcome, whereas the ones below were associated with reduced drinking (Monti, Rohsenow, Rubonis, Niaura, Sirota, Colby, Goddard, & Abrams, 1993; Rohsenow et al., 2001).

Passive Delay and Delay as a Cognitive Strategy

Passive Delay Procedure. During the first CET session, we ask clients simply to continue focusing on the beverage and reporting urges to "see what happens." With all of our clients, the urge began to decrease within 15 minutes of starting exposure. Some spontaneously began to use cognitive coping strategies; others found the drink boring when they continued to look at it without drinking. When their urge to drink is as low as they think it will go, or down to at least a 2 on the scale (many clients never get down to "No urge at all"), tell them they can stop focusing on the beverage. Ask them what they were thinking about, then discuss aspects that brought the urge up, and what they were thinking when the urge came down. Ask them if they had expected the urge to come down. Most of our clients said that they were sure that the urge to drink would never abate, and they were quite surprised when it went down to a manageable level so quickly. This disconfirmation of expectations may be the greatest benefit of having clients wait out the urge. They personally experience the fact that if they do nothing else, the urge will go down, so long as they do not drink.

Delay as a Cognitive Strategy. Immediately afterwards, we point out that the urges usually decrease if they wait long enough, but that people with drinking problems usually have never waited out a strong urge. This means that when they have an urge in the future, they can remind themselves that the urge will go down if they wait it out (e.g., "I can wait it out—no one ever died from an urge."). Without the personal experience, they would not believe this. We refer to waiting as an active coping self-instructional strategy, as the "Wait It Out" tool. After treatment, it is probably more useful when combined with other tools that can bring the urge down more rapidly, so in later sessions, we have them practice combining this with other tools.

Negative Consequences of Drinking

During the instructional phase, tell clients to list all the bad things that could happen to them if they were to take a drink after treatment. Although clients draw on past experiences, the focus is on the negative results that could occur in the future if they were to drink in the trigger situation when sober after treatment. Have them develop a list of fairly immediate negative consequences, then ask them to evaluate each consequence for its personal importance to them. Write this list on the Personal Toolbox. When you have them practice this strategy, either ask them to think about a specific consequence of their choice in the trigger situation or just tell them, "Think about all the bad things that would happen if you drank in that situation." Generally, some consequences work better in some situations than in others, and clients prefer to vary the ones on which they focus.

Clients generally already know how to think of the bad consequences that have happened to them, so this strategy comes easily. The difference is to have them focus on future negative consequences rather than only on past ones. For example, a client has already lost his wife, so that won't happen again when using this skill during the next 6 months, but he might fear losing his new job (one he never had before, so it was not a negative consequence in the past).

Positive Consequences of Sobriety

When instructing clients in this strategy, ask them to list all the positive things that could happen to them if they were to refrain from drinking when tempted. It is important that they focus on future positive consequences rather than just putting "not" before negative consequences. This is difficult for many clients; they are not used to thinking about what they have to gain from sobriety, and this is a strength of this strategy. Again, ask them to evaluate each consequence for its personal importance to them and write this list in their Personal Toolbox. In practicing this strategy, ask them either to think about a specific consequence or set of consequences that they think would help them in the specific trigger situation, or just tell them, "Think about all the good things that would happen if you stayed sober in that situation." Again, some consequences work better in some situations than in others, and clients prefer to vary the ones on which they focus.

Alternative Food or Drink

Clients are asked to generate a list of beverages or foods that give them pleasure and that they can obtain easily in some of their trigger situations; these are listed in their toolbox. Two types of trigger situations lend themselves to this strategy: (1) a social gathering at someone else's house, and (2) when clients are bored or stressed at home (e.g., watching TV or coming home from work).

Alternative Behaviors

Ask clients to generate a list of alternative activities that they could easily engage in without much advance notice that would be effective in distracting them from their urge to drink. If the trigger involves a negative mood, the activity should involve pleasure, or give a sense of accomplishment, or include social support. Be wary of activities that involve driving, since many clients drive automatically to the liquor store. Activities that cannot be engaged in within an hour will not be effective, such as the trip to India one client proposed.

INDIVIDUAL DIFFERENCES IN CUE REACTIVITY

Responders versus Nonresponders to Beverage Cues or Imaginal Cues

Using our standardized cue reactivity assessment methods, we have found across studies that about one-third of alcoholic clients do not respond to the beverage cues with increased urge to drink (relative to the neutral beverage) and about one-fourth to one-third of clients do not respond with elevated salivation. There may be several explanations for the lack of urge in response to beverage cues, including resistance to experiencing urges, experiencing urges but failing to report them due to a desire to present a socially desirable front, or the fact that it is not the beverage that makes them drink so much as emotional or social experiences.

Similarly, in CET sessions, some clients do not report increased urge when looking at the beverage cues. However, because the therapist has a chance to work through clients' sources of resistance to experiencing urges, fewer clients report no urge during CET. Because increased urge and increased salivation are independent of each other, someone who does not report elevations in urge may still respond with increased salivation or other physiological reactions. For this reason, those who continue to report no urge in response to the beverage are still exposed to the beverage for a set period of time during each session. We chose 8 minutes, because it is the average length of time it took responders to decrease their level of urge to at least a 2 on the urge scale.

We find that very few clients fail to respond to any of the imaginal scenes with elevated reports of urge. When nonresponse occurs, it is generally because clients are deliberately blocking their responses, and they can usually be encouraged to let themselves feel their urge. Rarely, we may encounter someone who has difficulty with imaging, so that the therapist may need to narrate the scene. More often, we find the opposite: Some clients expect that nothing will give them an urge to drink anymore and are surprised when scenes have the power to evoke urges. This helps to break through denial and motivate them to work more seriously on their total treatment program.

The Role of Affect in Cue Reactivity

While much of our research on alcohol cue reactivity has emphasized the sight and smell of beverage cues (exteroceptive stimuli), because they are the final common pathways before drinking, affective states can also play a strong role in cue reactivity. First, affective states may provide interoceptive stimuli to which cue reactivity became conditioned when drinking alcohol was repeatedly paired with the affective states. Second, negative affective states may increase the intensity of urges by increasing the salience of the desired immediate positive effects of alcohol. Analyses of relapse have found that a majority of alcohol relapses reported by alcoholics occurred in an interpersonal or intrapersonal negative mood state (Marlatt & Gordon, 1980).

Several studies found that the stronger the client's reported negative mood prior to exposure to beverage cues, the greater the urge to drink in response to the cues (Greeley, Swift, & Heather, 1992; Rohsenow et al., 1992). Although depression and anxiety correlated significantly with cue-elicited urge to drink, these measures were not significantly related to salivation, a physiological indicator of cue reactivity (Rohsenow et al., 1992).

A few studies have manipulated negative affect through the use of guided imagery procedures that provide a practical way to deliver substance use cues that elevate affect (Cooney et al., 1997). In the first such study, 8 alcoholic patients were exposed to hypnotic inductions of negative affect states that had been associated with drinking and were then exposed to the sight and smell of their preferred alcoholic beverage (Litt et al., 1990). In this small sample, negative mood induction was sufficient to elicit desire to drink, with no additional effect of the beverage. However, the hypnotic induction procedure, because it included deep relaxation, may have interfered with the effects of beverage exposure. In a second study, 57 alcoholic inpatients were exposed to a neutral beverage, then to an alcohol beverage, then to a description of a negative mood situation that the individual associated with drinking, and then another exposure to the alcohol beverage (Rubonis et al., 1994). Whereas beverage exposure alone increased urge to drink equally for both men and women, the negative mood induction further increased urge to drink only among the women, suggesting that women may be more susceptible to negative mood states as drinking triggers. In a third study with the same design, urge to drink was higher in the alcohol trial after the mood induction than the alcohol trial before mood induction for 68 alcoholic patients, of whom 72% were men, whereas salivation decreased across the same alcohol trials (Monti et al., 1999). In a fourth study, 50 male, alcoholic inpatients were presented a guided imagery description of either a neutral- or a negative-mood situation, based on the negative mood they had identified as most associated with drinking (Cooney et al., 1997). Then, they were exposed to both a neutral beverage and an alcohol beverage, in counterbalanced order. The mood induction and the alcohol beverage presentation each independently increased the patients' desire to drink and decreased their confidence that they could resist drinking. The alcohol beverage presentation, but not the mood induction, also resulted in increased heart rate and skin conductance levels compared to the neutral beverage condition. Thus, although alcohol beverage exposure alone results in increased urge to drink for most alcoholic patients, inducing a negative mood that is personally associated with drinking can also increase urge to drink, either alone or in combination with beverage exposure. These studies provide support for the use of both beverage cues and guided imagery of mood states in the exposure sessions.

Alcohol Dependence and Cue Reactivity

One question is whether cue reactivity levels are greater for those with higher levels of alcohol dependence. In two studies that conducted standardized cue reactivity assessment, scores on the Alcohol Dependence Scale (Skinner & Allen, 1982) correlated with increased levels of salivation and urge to drink in one study but not the other study (Rohsenow et al., 1992). The Rand study's measure of alcohol dependence (Polich, Armor, & Braiker, 1981) had no correlation with either desire to drink or changes in heart rate or skin conductance in response to cues in a third study (Cooney et al., 1997). A measure of severity of alcohol dependence correlated significantly with a composite measure of reactivity to alcohol cues in another study (Glautier & Drummond, 1994). Therefore, cue reactivity may be greater at times among persons with greater alcohol dependence. However, CET is conducted the same, regardless of degree of dependence.

FORM 5.1. Drinking Triggers Interview

Part 1: ELICIT TRIGGERS

"I'd like you to list for me the triggers [that is, situations or events] that were frequently associated with heavy drinking for you in the past year." Have clients be specific. Probe for most common environments, people, and feelings while drinking.

A client may think that we're asking him/her what *caused* the drinking and may feel unable to answer for that reason. If this is a problem, clarify it. "We are not asking about causes; instead we want to know any situations or events where you drank a lot or any situations that led to a strong urge to drink."

Prompts:

"What most often triggered or set off a drinking bout for you?"

"What was happening when you had your last drinking bout?"

"What are some other situations where you might have a strong urge to drink, or where you would have trouble resisting drinking?"

"Is drinking heavily associated with any specific *places* for you?" (such as: bars, work settings, certain houses)

"Were you more likely to drink heavily when you were *feeling bad*?" (such as: angry, depressed, worried, uptight, frustrated, lonely, bored, guilty, under a lot of pressure)

"Were you more likely to drink heavily when you had *problems with other people* or you felt tense or uneasy around other people?"

"Were you more likely to drink heavily when you were *feeling good*?"

"Were you more likely to drink heavily when you were with other *people who drank*?"

"Were you more likely to drink heavily when you saw something like a bottle or a bar that *reminded you of drinking*?" (examples: like a bottle or can of your usual drink, an advertisement, a liquor store, the outside of a bar)

"Were you more likely to drink heavily when you were *feeling sick, jumpy, or tired*?" (such as: in pain, to stay awake, to get to sleep, stomach upset or in knots)

Part 2: OBTAIN URGE, AFFECT, AND FREQUENCY INFORMATION

A. Explain the "urge" concept:
"While you are participating in this treatment, you will be asked to rate your urge to drink in different situations. By urge, we mean how much craving, wish, desire, or thirst to drink you have, whether or not you intend to drink."

For each trigger, ask: "If you were in this situation today, how much would your urge to drink be?" Show the client a card with the urge scale (use upper half of Figure 5.1) on it, and ask him/her to answer on a 0–10 scale. This card is referred to as the "urge card."

B. Confidence ratings:
For each trigger, ask: "If you were in this situation today, how confident are you that you would not drink?" Show the client a card with the confidence scale on it, and ask the client to rate his/her answer on the 0–10 scale. (Use lower half of Figure 5.1.)

C. Rank-order triggers for frequency:
Ask: "Which of these triggers most often happens just before you drink? Which is most often associated with drinking for you?"

(continued)

Construct a hierarchy of the triggers by rank-ordering in terms of "urge to drink" in each situation. Break any ties by ranking more frequent situations higher.

DRINKING TRIGGERS ANSWER SHEET

Trigger number	Write triggers here. Draw a line between each trigger.	Urge	Conf.	How often?

FORM 5.2. Urge-Specific Strategies Questionnaire

Actual Strategies:

When you have an urge to drink, what do you do to try to keep yourself from drinking?

What else do you do? [ASK "WHAT ELSE?" UNTIL NO MORE ANSWERS ARE GIVEN.]

IF SUBJECT SAYS HE/SHE DOESN'T TRY TO RESIST THE URGE, ASK: Did you ever try to resist the urge to drink, even on the first day you left treatment, or at least once in the last 6 months?

	(show scale cards)	
Draw a line between each strategy:	How Often	How Effective

(continued)

When you have an urge to drink, and are trying to keep yourself from drinking, how *often* do you . . .

When you have an urge to drink, and are trying to keep yourself from drinking, how *effective* do you think it is to . . .

	How Often	How Effective
tell yourself that if you just wait awhile, the urge to drink will go down?	_____	_____
think about the bad things that would happen if you drank?	_____	_____
think about the good things you have in your life by staying sober?	_____	_____
use imagery to cope with the urge; for example, do you imagine the urge is like a wave that builds up and then fades away, or imagine stomping on the urge, or imagine using a weapon to cut down the urge to drink?	_____	_____
try to eat or drink something other than alcohol?	_____	_____
find something you can do instead of drinking alcohol that would help to reduce the urge to drink?	_____	_____
tell yourself mastery messages, like "I can take charge of this urge," or "I am not going to let this urge win"?	_____	_____
try to distract yourself somehow; for example, do you try to imagine that you are somewhere else that's calm and quiet, like a beach or forest or some other special place?	_____	_____
try to use relaxation techniques, to relax the muscles in your body?	_____	_____
try to use meditation techniques, to empty out your mind of all bad thoughts?	_____	_____
try to get away from the situation that is giving you an urge to drink?	_____	_____

USSQ RATING SCALES

How often have you tried this when you had an urge to drink?

0	1	2	3	4	5	6	7	8	9	10
Never					Half the time					Every time

How effective was this?

0	1	2	3	4	5	6	7	8	9	10
Never stops me					Stops me about half the time					Always stops me

154

Therapist Tip Sheet: Cue Exposure Treatment Rationale

1. In treatment, your urges or cravings for alcohol will go down.
   - Because you are away from triggers (people, places, things associated with drinking).
   - But urges may return after you leave the program.
   - Learning to handle urges here will make you better prepared for later.
2. It's best to avoid triggers but you can't avoid all triggers when you leave the program.
   - Ads on TV, a party with drinks, feelings of anger or loneliness.
3. The purpose of this treatment is to help you learn how to reduce your urge to drink while you are in a safe place. The treatment works by having you:
   - Experience triggers until you feel your urges decrease.
   - Learn and practice specific coping skills to bring your urges down.
   - Some skills you already know, others will be new.
4. Don't expose yourself to triggers on your own.
   - It's not safe without counselor support.
   - The goal is to help you handle triggers you can't avoid; it's not to make you able to expose yourself to risk.
5. Each session begins with exposure to your typical drink. Then you will imagine being in high-risk situations.
   - First, you will focus your attention just on the drink or situation.
   - Later, you will practice using coping skills.
6. With practice, handling urges will get easier. You will be prepared for when you run into a trigger situation outside of treatment,
   - You will learn that your urges go away without drinking.
   - You will learn which coping skills work best for you.
   - You will use coping skills more quickly and effectively.

Therapist Tip Sheet: CET Individual Session 1

PREPARATION

1. Get Tip Sheet, individual's DTI form, urge and confidence display cards, clock or stopwatch, tissues to deal with spills.
2. Bring beverage and glass to treatment room in enclosed cooler. Place cooler out of view until ready for use.

STARTING THE SESSION

1. Review *Rationale*, solicit questions.
2. Complete *DTI* form (if not done prior to session).
3. Review concept of urge (want, wish, desire, thirst for). Introduce, explain *urge card*.
4. Explain *urge monitoring* to subject (e.g., tell me if it changes; give me a number; your use of a timer). Anytime urge changes, record new urge level and time.

ALCOHOL EXPOSURE

1. *Starting the exposure*

   "Now I'm going to bring out the drinks. During this time I want you to let yourself feel the urge as fully as possible, to experience the urge as it builds and see what happens to it. During this time, I would like you not to use any coping tools, but simply to experience the urge. Tell me every time your urge changes—give me a number."

   "Now I'd like you to pour your drink in the glass. Only fill it about halfway. I would like you to hold the glass or bottle all the time, and keep looking at it. Notice the aspects that give you the strongest urge—whether it is the sight, the smell, the feeling of the glass/bottle/can, and focus on these aspects. Let me know when the urge is as high as you think it will go. Are you ready to begin?"

   Start the stopwatch, bring bottle/can, then glass out. Have client prepare his/her drink.

   Prompts:

   "Continue to focus *just* on the [beverage] and whatever it is about the [beverage] that makes you want it, whether it's the way it makes you *feel*, the *smell*, the *taste*, *holding* it, the *label*, the *bottle*, etc."

   (continued)

"I want you to think about *nothing* else. Just let yourself experience the urge. This is a safe place. Stay with it and just see what happens."

2. *At maximum urge* (either a 10 *or* when urge starts decreasing *or* when client states urge is at its ceiling), say, **"OK, I think it's reached as high as it's going to go. Let's see what happens if you just keep looking at it and holding it. Tell me whenever your urge changes."** Monitor urge changes and time until urge is as low as it can go, but at least a 2 or lower. Then say, **"OK, you can stop thinking about the drink now."**

   If no urge, explore barriers:
   a. *Thoughts.* What thoughts? Correct errors (e.g., imagining drinking).
   b. *Unwilling to feel urge.* Emphasize importance, the safety.

   "It's important to let yourself experience the urge. We know that people who are aware of their urges and their reactions do better, are better able to cope."

   c. *Reassure.* **"You may still be having reactions that you're not aware of, like higher heart rate, saliva, blood pressure. These reactions will be affected by the exposure anyway."**

3. *Discuss the exposure experience.* Assess spontaneous use of any coping tools during exposure: **"What were you thinking? Did you try to do anything to bring the urge down? How did this compare to what you expected to happen?"**

4. *Teach first tool.* Delay: The "Wait It Out" tool. Impress upon the client how the urge went down by waiting it out. That he/she can tell self in future that urge will go down if he/she doesn't drink.

IMAGINAL EXPOSURE TO TRIGGER

1. *Leave beverage* in glass with bottle/can open. Say that the client can close eyes if it helps him/her.

2. *Start trigger scene exposure.*

   "In a minute I'll ask you to imagine the _____ trigger [highest ranked one]. I want you to put yourself in the situation, imagine it fully, feel an urge. Later I will ask you to practice using your tool, but don't do it until then. I don't want you to imagine yourself drinking, but instead get to the point where you desire a drink, by just focusing on whatever it is about the trigger that makes you want to drink. Imagine what you see, hear, smell, and feel in that situation. OK? Imagine you are . . . [describe trigger fully]."

   Start stopwatch. Prompt as needed. Reinforce signs of affect.

(continued)

3. *At maximum urge* (either a 10 *or* when urge starts decreasing *or* when client states urge is at its ceiling) say, **"OK, now, let's see what happens. Be sure to tell me whenever your urge changes."** Monitor urge changes and time until urge is at 2 or below. Then terminate scene. **"OK, you can stop thinking about that situation."**

4. *Discuss the exposure* experience. Assess any spontaneous use of any coping tools during exposure: **"What were you thinking?"** Discuss any effects of simple delay—**"How did this compare to what you expected to happen?"**

5. *Repeat scene* using the **"Wait It Out"** tool as an active coping strategy. When urge is at maximum, say, **"Now imagine staying where you are but telling yourself that if you just wait it out, the urge will go down."**

   Terminate and discuss as before. Ask whether this tool helps. Point out if urge decreased more quickly when using this tool.

SESSION TERMINATION

1. Discuss *reactions* to session.
2. Prepare client for *urges outside of treatment* session. Encourage *practice* of coping tools if urge is encountered outside of treatment session. Prohibit practice of exposure, but encourage practice of tools.
3. *Assess urge*; talk down elevated urge if necessary before allowing client to leave the building. Methods: Encourage client to use any coping tool, or distract him/her from urge by discussing irrelevant subject.

Therapist Tip Sheet: CET Individual Sessions after First Session

STARTING THE SESSION

1. *Check in.* Deal with issues.
2. Add any *new drinking triggers* and assess urge, confidence, and frequency in new trigger situation.

ALCOHOL EXPOSURE

1. *Starting the exposure*

   "Now I'm going to bring out the drinks. During this time, I want you to let yourself feel the urge as fully as possible. I would like you not to use any coping tools until I tell you to, but simply to experience the urge.

   "Now I'd like you to pour your drink [only half full]. **Hold the glass or bottle all the time, and keep looking at it. Notice the aspects that give you the strongest urge— whether it is the sight, the smell, the feeling of the glass/can/bottle, and focus on these aspects. Are you ready to begin?"**

   Start the stopwatch, bring bottle/can, then glass out. Have client prepare his/her drink.

   Prompts:

   "Continue to focus *just* on the [beverage] and whatever it is about the [beverage] that makes you want it, whether it's the way it makes you *feel*, the *smell*, the *taste*, *holding* it, the *label*, the *bottle*, etc."

   "I want you to think about *nothing* else. Just let yourself experience the urge. This is a safe place. Stay with it and just see what happens."

2. *At maximum urge* say, **"OK, now use [the newest tool] to get the urge down. Be sure to tell me every time your urge changes."**

   Terminate beverage exposure when the urge is a 2 or less. **"OK, you can stop thinking about the drink now."**

3. *Discuss the exposure* experience. Assess use of any other coping tools during exposure, what they were thinking. Ask, **"What happened to the urge before and after using the tool?" "How well did this tool work?"**

   (continued)

If urge went up, then came down:

a. *Change.* Comment on change in urge.
b. *Coping.* What happened? Which strategies? How well did or didn't they work?
c. *Matching tools to triggers.* Which tool works better with this particular trigger?
d. *Spontaneous strategies.* Reinforce, record them on the toolbox.
e. *Enhance self-efficacy.* Reinforce any success, and not drinking despite an urge.

If no urge experienced:

Discuss *barriers* to experience.
Encourage client to let him/herself experience an urge so that he/she can feel the power of the coping strategies.

4. *Introduce type of coping strategy.*

   a. *Describe today's coping tool.* **"Now we're going to talk about . . . "**
   b. *Personalize it*: Have client describe his/her most salient personal strategies or examples for that skill type.
   c. *Write on the toolbox form*: have client write down his/her personal examples.
   d. *List of tools*
      • Delay and "Wait It Out" (first session).
      • Think about the bad things that would happen if you drank.
      • Think about the good things that would happen if you stayed sober.
      • Eat or drink something else.
      • Do something else.

5. *Repeat beverage exposure with* practice of new *tool.* First let urge go up without using tool, then when urge peaks say, **"Now I'd like you to use the [new tool] to bring your urge down."** Afterwards, explore how the tool was used and how well it worked.

IMAGINAL EXPOSURE TO TRIGGER

1. *Leave beverage* in glass with bottle/can open. Client can use beverage in imaginal exposure if that increases urge. Remind client to close eyes if he/she wants.

2. *Start trigger scene exposure, then add coping.*
   "In a minute I'll ask you to imagine the _____ trigger [highest ranked trigger]. I want you to put yourself in the situation, imagine it fully, feel an urge. At a certain point, I will ask you to practice using your tool, but don't do it until then. I don't want you to imagine yourself drinking, but instead get to the point where you would like to drink, by just focusing on whatever it is about the trigger that makes you want to drink. Imagine what you see, hear, smell, and feel in that situation. OK? Imagine you are . . . [describe trigger fully]."

   Start stopwatch. Prompt as needed. Reinforce signs of affect.

(continued)

3. *At maximum urge* say, **"OK, I want you to imagine staying where you are but now imagine using [the new tool] to get your urge down. Be sure to tell me any time your urge changes."** In later sessions, encourage subject to use **"any tool or combination of tools"** to reduce urge to drink, so client can practice thinking of the tools him/herself.

   Prompts:
   "Keep imagining you are in that situation but using [tool]."

   Terminate scene when urge is at least 2 or below. **"OK, you can stop thinking about that situation."**

4. *Discuss the exposure* experience. Ask what happened to the urge before and after using the tool. Assess use of directed and/or spontaneous coping tools during exposure, what were they thinking. **"How well did this tool work?"**

   If urge went up then came down:
   a. *Change.* Comment on change in urge.
   b. *Coping.* What happened? Which strategies? How well did or didn't they work?
   c. *Matching tools to triggers.* Which tool works better with this particular trigger?
   d. *Spontaneous strategies.* Reinforce, record them on the toolbox.
   e. *Enhance self-efficacy.* Reinforce any success, and not drinking despite an urge.

   If no urge experienced:

   Discuss *barriers* to experience.
   Encourage client to let him/herself experience an urge so that he/she can feel the power of the coping strategies.

5. *Repeat* with additional scenes. Over sessions, get through all triggers and do each trigger several times with different tools each time.

6. Ensure that all tools are tried with each of the major triggers. Discuss which tools work better for this person in each trigger situation in summary statements.

SESSION TERMINATION

1. Discuss *reactions* to session.
2. Prepare client for *urges outside of treatment* session. Encourage *practice* of coping tools if urge is encountered outside of treatment session. Prohibit practice of exposure.
3. *Assess urge* before leaving room; talk down elevated urge, if necessary.

LAST SESSION

1. *Review all tools.* Concentrate on client's own most effective ones for each type of trigger.
2. Remind that *escape or avoidance* is still the most effective first line of defense.
3. Give client copy of his/her own *personalized toolbox* (typed).

Reminder Sheet: _____'s Toolbox for Reducing Urges

1. **Things I can say to help me wait it out:**
   * _____
   * _____
   * _____
   * _____
   * _____

2. **Negative results if I started to drink again:**
   * _____
   * _____
   * _____
   * _____
   * _____
   * _____

3. **Positive results of sobriety for me:**
   * _____
   * _____
   * _____
   * _____
   * _____
   * _____

4. **Eat or drink something else:**
   * _____
   * _____
   * _____
   * _____
   * _____
   * _____

5. **Do something else:**
   * _____
   * _____
   * _____
   * _____

SIX

Dual Diagnosis Issues

General Introduction   163
Depression   166
Anxiety Disorders   168
Psychotic Disorders   169
Personality Disorders   171
Tobacco Dependence Issues   173

GENERAL INTRODUCTION

A high percentage of clients with alcohol or drug use disorders have a concomitant psychiatric disorder. Recent estimates (Rosenthal & Westreich, 1999) are that 37% of those with alcohol abuse/dependence and 53% of those with drug abuse/dependence also have psychiatric disorders, the most common of which are affective, anxiety, psychotic, and personality disorders. Among psychiatric patients, 20–50% have co-occurring alcohol or drug use disorders.

There are various possible etiologies for these co-occurring disorders: The substance use and psychiatric disorders may have independent etiologies; the substance use disorder may be secondary to the psychiatric disorder or vice versa; or both may be secondary to a common third factor (Meyer, 1986). Regardless of how they came about, once present, they may influence both the course of illness and the course of recovery of each other. For that reason, no treatment program focused primarily on either type of disorder in clients can ignore the possibility of the other.

Routine screening is therefore recommended to detect substance abuse problems among clients who present in psychiatric settings and psychiatric problems among clients who present in substance abuse settings. In psychiatric treatment settings, a combination of self-report screening questions, collateral information from friends or family, and biochem-

ical measures, such as urine and/or breath tests, are useful to detect alcohol or drug problems (Carey & Correia, 1998). Although many self-report substance abuse screening ques-
tionnaires are available, the Dartmouth Assessment of Lifestyle Instrument (DALI) is
recommended, because it was developed specifically for the identification of alcohol or
drug abuse in persons with severe mental illness (Rosenberg et al., 1998). In substance
abuse settings, the Psychiatric Severity subscale of the Addiction Severity Index (ASI;
McLellan et al., 1992) provides relatively brief screening for psychopathology. However,
Carey, Cocco, and Correia (1997) warn that the ASI subscales may have reduced reliability
and validity in clients with severe mental illness. We have found that self-administered ques-
tionnaires such as the Beck Depression Inventory (Beck, Ward, Mendelson, Mock, &
Erbaugh, 1961) and the State–Trait Anxiety Inventory (Spielberger, Gorsuch, & Lushene,
1970), given at several points during the course of treatment, are useful for identifying and
tracking problematic symptoms.

The process of making a psychiatric diagnosis is complicated by the fact that one may
be unable to discriminate between substance-induced symptoms and symptoms of a true
psychiatric disorder (e.g., Schuckit et al., 1997). A single diagnostic interview conducted
early in abstinence is likely to be unreliable, but, unfortunately, agreement has yet to be
achieved regarding the length of abstinence required before an accurate psychiatric diagnosis can be made. Drake and colleagues (1990) recommend a consensus approach for diag-
nosing substance use disorders in persons with severe mental illness, combining self-report
and interview data, along with collateral reports and longitudinal data accumulated by case
managers, through repeated contacts over time.

Another consideration in the assessment of clients with dual psychiatric and substance
use disorders is determination of their readiness to change either disorder. Ziedonis and
Trudeau (1997) found that about half of dually diagnosed outpatients in a mental health
clinic were only in the precontemplation or contemplation stages of change for their substance abuse. Most of the treatment procedures described in this volume are geared to individuals in an action stage of change, so a motivational enhancement intervention (e.g.,
Miller & Rollnick, 2002) may be a prerequisite to attempting coping skills training for many
dual diagnosis patients. Several self-report measures for assessing readiness to change
are available, such as the University of Rhode Island Change Assessment (URICA;
DiClemente & Hughes, 1990) or the Stages of Change Readiness and Treatment Eagerness
Scale (SOCRATES; Miller & Tonigan, 1996). The Substance Abuse Treatment Scale (SATS;
McHugo, Drake, Burton, & Ackerson, 1995) was specifically designed to describe psychiatric patients' stage (among eight possibilities) in the process of recovery from substance use
disorders.

With respect to treatment for co-occurring substance use and psychiatric disorders,
some interventions that may be utilized focus exclusively on one or the other type of disorder (e.g., medications, such as antidepressants, antianxiety agents, anticraving drugs; or
suggesting that clients attend AA). However, a number of psychosocial interventions can
benefit both types of disorder. For example, because negative moods or anger are aspects
of some psychiatric disorders and are also frequent relapse precipitants, interventions that
focus on identifying and managing negative moods and/or anger will likely contribute to
improvements in both the psychiatric and substance use disorders. Similarly, lack of social
support may be an obstacle to recovery from both psychiatric and substance use disorders,

and both conditions are likely to be improved by providing training in social skills and effective communication. Other skills training interventions that may be beneficial for both types of disorder include problem solving, stress management, increasing pleasant activities, and vocational rehabilitation.

Beyond consideration of beneficial interventions for co-occurring disorders, the manner of their delivery must be adapted for these challenging clients. Providing a high degree of structure, with clearly stated ground rules that are consistently enforced, can serve to compensate for lack of internal controls among dual diagnosis clients. Keeping explanations of new skills at a simple level, breaking them down into small steps, providing concrete examples of their application, and engaging in considerable practice can help to compensate for cognitive limitations. Dual diagnosis clients can be especially reactive to confrontation and pressure imposed by therapists and will therefore be more likely to remain in treatment if their comfort level is maintained by avoiding direct confrontations. Therapists are advised to adopt a "coaching" style, in which they join with the client to work together toward mutually agreed-upon goals.

Drake (1996) emphasized that recovery among severe dual diagnosis clients is typically a protracted affair, often developing gradually over a period of years. As a result, there needs to be greater tolerance for lapses back to substance use, utilizing them as opportunities to learn more about relapse triggers and to develop better means of avoiding or coping with the triggers. Along similar lines, Carey (1996) has advocated the inclusion of a harm reduction philosophy when working with dual diagnosis clients in outpatient psychiatric treatment. Her comprehensive, five-point program includes establishing a working alliance with the client; evaluating the costs and benefits of the client's substance use; identifying client goals for change (with therapist willingness to accept a nonabstinent goal as a means of reducing substance-related harm), building a lifestyle and environment that support recovery; and developing plans for coping with crises.

A final general issue to consider in working with dual diagnosis clients relates to the optimal sequencing and/or combining of the psychiatric and chemical dependence aspects of treatment. Typically, substance abuse treaters believe that effective treatment cannot begin until the acute psychiatric symptoms are dealt with, and mental health professionals often feel that nothing can be accomplished as long as the client is actively using alcohol or drugs. Actually, because both psychiatric and chemical dependence problems are typically disruptive, and improvements in them are often gradual, one does not have the luxury of waiting for one disorder to stabilize before treating the other. Therefore, the acute manifestations of both must be addressed in parallel. Fortunately, improvement in one often makes improvement in the other more likely.

If a client poses an imminent danger to self or others, this obviously needs to be attended to immediately. Beyond that, however, initial treatment efforts should be directed toward reducing or eliminating both the substance use and the most disruptive psychiatric symptoms, followed by sustained efforts to address the remaining salient aspects of both problems in parallel. In the ideal situation, both types of problem would be addressed by the same set of treaters. However, if each is addressed independently by a different specialist, then careful attention must be paid to maintaining ongoing communication and coordination between them, to maximize their synergy and reduce the stress on clients of having multiple treaters, and the associated possibility of treatment dropout. During the course of treatment, there should be open discussion of psychiatric symptoms, use of medications, and involvement of other professionals. This will minimize clients' splitting of their various caregivers and avoid stigmatizing their psychiatric problems, which would prevent clients from discussing them and learning about their connection to substance use. It is important for providers working primarily on substance abuse issues to have a detailed understanding of the concurrent pharmacological treatment that has been prescribed and to monitor adherence to the medication regimen, because the effects of noncompliance can be a potent trigger for relapse to substance use. Although the controlled environment of a hospital inpatient unit, or a residential setting, would provide the greatest structure and safety for initiating pharmacological interventions, these settings are not likely to be accessible except for the most severe psychiatric disorders or when clients exhibit acute possibility of danger to self or others.

Having covered some general principles regarding interventions with dual diagnosis clients, we now turn to the use of cognitive-behavioral techniques in the context of specific comorbid disorders. The following sections of this chapter describe interventions and resource material aimed primarily at the psychiatric disorders that commonly co-occur with substance use disorders. However, it is relatively rare that co-occurring psychiatric and substance use disorders are so clearly differentiated that they can be treated totally independently of one another. Typically, there are varying degrees of interaction between them, and interventions intended to affect one also impact the other.

DEPRESSION

Depression is among the most prevalent of co-occurring disorders, and indicates poor prognosis and increased likelihood of dropout from treatment for chemical dependence (Brown, Evans, Miller, Burgess, & Mueller, 1997). Marlatt and Gordon (1985) reported that negative moods are the most common precipitant of relapse, a finding that has been replicated across a number of studies. However, it is difficult to sort out cause and effect for comorbid depression, because alcohol-induced depression presents very similarly to independently occurring depression (Kadden, Kranzler, & Rounsaville, 1995; Raimo & Schuckit, 1998). The distinction has treatment implications, because alcohol-induced depressive states in the first week of treatment are often significantly reduced by the second week, without intervention (Brown & Schuckit, 1988).

Cognitive-behavioral interventions have demonstrated efficacy for the treatment of depression, and have revealed more enduring effects than pharmacotherapy, possibly because they address factors that contribute to risk, and/or because clients acquire skills that enable them to cope with high-risk situations (Hollon & Beck, 1994). Parenthetically, there has been some interest in the impact of pharmacotherapies intended for depression on the occurrence of drinking. However, these studies have had mixed results, with some reporting beneficial effects of medication (e.g., Cornelius et al., 1997), and others showing no effect on drinking despite improvement in depression (e.g., McGrath et al., 1996).

Brown et al. (1997) described a cognitive-behavioral intervention for depressed alcoholics that had its origins in a treatment manual for coping with depression (Brown & Lewinsohn, 1984), in rational–emotive therapy (Ellis & Harper, 1961), and in methods for identifying cognitive distortions (Beck, Rush, Shaw, & Emery, 1979). The intervention involves educating clients about the reciprocal relationships among behavior, thoughts, and mood, as well as between depressive symptoms and alcohol use. A rationale is provided for utilizing coping skills to control depressive symptoms that might otherwise serve as triggers to drink. In fact, the coping skills are similar to those commonly used to deal with other triggers for drinking. Specific interventions include asking clients to make daily ratings of their moods, along with associated events and thoughts. As they become more aware of their emotions and related thoughts, cognitive techniques are employed to increase positive thoughts, decrease negative thoughts, and identify and dispute cognitive distortions. Social and communication skills training are provided to cope with social pressure to drink, as well as with conflicts that are often followed by drinking and/or depression. Clients are encouraged to increase pleasurable activities to prevent the onset of depressive symptoms. Maintenance strategies are also taught, including ongoing monitoring of moods and strategies to prevent or manage depressed moods. Brown et al. (1997) found that the addition of this training package to a treatment program resulted in greater reductions in subjects' depressive symptoms, better drinking outcomes, and superior maintenance of these effects compared to a control group.

The Project MATCH Cognitive-Behavioral Coping Skills Therapy Manual (Kadden et al., 1992), based to a large extent on the first edition of this treatment guide, also addresses the problem of depression among alcoholics. It does so through an added session on managing negative moods and depression, based largely on the work of Emery (1981). Specific steps are outlined for developing awareness of the presence of negative thoughts and symptoms of depression, each instance of which is treated as a separate problem to be solved. Typical distortions of thinking are identified, along with a considerable number of techniques that can be helpful in correcting the distortions. In addition to cognitive interventions, a number of actions are suggested to challenge automatic negative thoughts, including problem solving to cope with issues that cause worry or concern, increasing pleasant activities, and decreasing unpleasant activities.

In their volume on the application of cognitive therapy to the problem of substance abuse, Beck, Wright, Newman, and Liese (1993) consider various psychiatric disorders that are most likely to co-occur with substance abuse. They provide information on identifying and modifying negatively biased cognitions, as well as suggestions for modifying automatic thoughts, such as cognitive rehearsal, diversion techniques, and organizing a schedule of activities. With respect to depression, they recommend that attention be paid to cognitive, affective, physiological, motivational, and behavioral symptoms, and they outline a multi-faceted therapeutic approach to deal with them.

There are a number of client self-help manuals for coping with depression. The one by Greenberger and Padesky (1995) provides exercises on identification of moods, challenging automatic thoughts, balanced thinking, cognitive restructuring, and improving interpersonal relationships and social support. The client manual by Lewinsohn, Munoz, Youngren, and Zeiss (1986) provides self-instruction in the areas of pleasant activities, social skills, and thought control.

Whether working with materials designed primarily for dually diagnosed clients or those targeted specifically at depression, there is enough similarity in the cognitive-behavioral interventions that are effective with both conditions that it is quite easy and natural to integrate them for use with depressed alcoholic clients. Cognitive-behavioral interventions most commonly employed with depressed alcoholics include the following:

- Increasing awareness of negative thoughts, depressive symptoms, and their relation to alcohol use; refuting cognitive distortions (e.g., managing negative thinking; anger management; receiving criticism).
- Developing skills to cope with various negative situations (problem solving).
- Organizing a schedule of pleasant activities (increasing pleasant activities).
- Improving interpersonal skills and enhancing social support (e.g., assertiveness, conversation skills, giving and receiving positive feedback, developing social support networks).

These interventions are described elsewhere in this volume, as well as in many other sources on the treatment of dual diagnosis clients.

Even among alcoholics who are not clinically depressed, there is often a fair amount of alcohol-induced depressive symptomatology in the early recovery period. These symptoms typically respond to the same cognitive-behavioral interventions employed with more depressed clients, and may also respond to the cognitive-behavioral interventions employed to treat the drinking problem itself.

ANXIETY DISORDERS

Substance use disorders commonly co-occur with anxiety disorders such as panic disorder, generalized anxiety disorder, social phobia, obsessive–compulsive disorder, and posttraumatic stress disorder (PTSD) (Deas-Nesmith, Brady, & Myrick, 1998). As with other comorbid psychiatric disorders, it is difficult to diagnose anxiety disorders in the context of active substance abuse. There is considerable overlap in the symptoms of anxiety disorders and those associated with substance intoxication and withdrawal. A primary anxiety disorder should be diagnosed only when symptoms of anxiety persist during several months of abstinence (Anthenelli & Schuckit, 1993).

Cognitive-behavioral techniques known to be effective in the treatment of both anxiety and substance use disorders include coping skills training, social skills training, cognitive restructuring, and cue exposure (see Barlow & Lehman, 1996, for a review of research on effective treatments for anxiety disorders). Mastery of anxiety symptoms through the use of coping skills may also help boost clients' confidence that their efforts to cope with addiction will be successful. In addition, learning anxiety-reducing coping skills may help clients to break out of the mind-set of using external agents to combat uncomfortable subjective states, thereby reducing the likelihood of relapse to substance use.

As noted earlier, Beck has adapted his approach to cognitive therapy for depression and anxiety to the treatment of substance abuse (Beck et al., 1993). This treatment model is well suited for work with dual disordered clients, using a variety of techniques to help clients deal with problems leading to emotional distress, and better understand their reliance on alcohol/drugs for pleasure or relief of discomfort. Specific cognitive strategies are taught to reduce urges and cravings, and more general cognitive therapy techniques are used to help clients combat depression, anxiety, or anger, which may serve as triggers for addictive behaviors. The use of this approach for dual diagnosis patients is supported by findings that cognitive therapy was more effective than drug counseling among methadone-maintained opioid addicts with higher levels of psychiatric severity (Woody et al., 1984).

In addition to cognitive and cognitive-behavioral therapies, various forms of pharmacological treatment can be effective for anxiety disorders. However, there is a potential for abuse of the commonly prescribed benzodiazepine medications in individuals with dual disorders. Agents with little or no abuse potential should be considered the first line of pharmacological treatment in this population (Deas-Nesmith et al., 1998).

To our knowledge, there is no published, controlled outcome study examining cognitive-behavioral treatment for individuals with both anxiety and substance use disorders, but the clinical literature contains several models of integrated treatment specifically for clients with both PTSD and substance abuse diagnoses. Meisler (1999) describes an outpatient group approach that includes psychoeducation about PTSD and substance abuse, instruction in sleep hygiene, motivational enhancement, and coping skills training in problem solving, relaxation, anger management, self-reinforcement, cognitive refocusing, assertiveness, drink refusal, receiving criticism, and enhancing social support. Meisler suggests that therapeutic exposure to both trauma and alcohol cues can be applied in the later phases of treatment. Abueg and Fairbank (1992) describe a model for staged treatment based on motivational readiness. It combines direct therapeutic exposure to trauma cues, problem solving, and relapse prevention coping skills, such as identification of high-risk relapse situations, enhancing social supports, cognitive techniques to managing negative emotions, substance cue exposure (using imagery), and drink refusal training. We have excluded patients with PTSD diagnoses from our alcohol cue exposure treatment, because reliving the trauma cues can be overwhelming to therapist and patient alike in that context. Specialized treatment for PTSD per se needs to be conducted with these clients in order to deal adequately with the role of trauma cues in alcohol relapse.

In summary, the recommendations for adapting substance abuse treatment to clients with comorbid alcohol dependence and anxiety disorders are as follows:

- Emphasizing general cognitive therapy sessions (managing negative thinking, anger management, problem solving).
- Emphasizing social skills useful for social phobia (e.g., conversational skills, nonverbal behavior, assertiveness, developing social support networks, drink refusal skills).
- Cue exposure with urge-specific coping skills training.
- Exposure therapy utilizing anxiety-provoking cues (e.g., systematic desensitization).
- Avoiding use of medications with abuse potential.

PSYCHOTIC DISORDERS

Substance use disorders are more prevalent among individuals with severe mental disorders than in the general population. According to the Epidemiologic Catchment Area Survey (Regier et al., 1990), 47% of persons with schizophrenia and 56% of persons with bipolar disorder have a lifetime diagnosis of substance abuse or dependence. This compares with a rate of 16% in the U.S. population. The high base rate of alcohol and drug abuse among individuals with severe mental illness (SMI) indicates that these individuals often need substance abuse services.

Substance abuse coping skills training as described in this book can be an important component in a comprehensive biopsychosocial treatment program for individuals with comorbid schizophrenia and alcohol or drug problems. Indeed, the skills training approach of this guide was first applied to the treatment of clients with SMI (Monti, Corriveau, & Curran, 1982a). In addition to coping skills training, these individuals may also require antipsychotic medication, assertive case management, and money management. Cognitive impairments and difficulties with attention, memory, and reality orientation may reduce patients' ability to benefit from coping skills training if it emphasizes cognitive changes. Ziedonis and D'Avanzo (1998) recommend that cognitive-behavioral therapy with substance abusers with schizophrenia be more behaviorally than cognitively focused.

Robert Drake (see, e.g., Drake, Bartels, Teague, Noordsy, & Clark, 1993) describes a general treatment approach for substance-abusing patients with SMI, emphasizing the need to deliver stagewise treatment to ensure the appropriate timing of substance abuse interventions. It begins with developing a trusting relationship or working alliance with the patient (engagement), followed by efforts to help the patient perceive the negative consequences of substance use (persuasion), achieve recovery (active treatment), and, in the final stage, maintain a stable recovery (relapse prevention). Coping skills training is most appropriate in the active treatment and relapse prevention stages of treatment.

A manual for group treatment of substance abusing patients with SMI has been developed based on Drake's model (Mueser, Fox, Kenison, & Geltz, 1995). A "better living skills" group is used to teach clients adaptive strategies for managing interpersonal situations, negative affective states, and leisure time, as well as to provide them with basic information about the effects of substance abuse and the interaction between substance abuse and psychiatric disorders. Session outlines are provided for the following topics: conversational skills, dealing with angry feelings, stress management, drink/drug refusal skills, coping with negative thoughts and feelings, and recreational and leisure activities.

Roberts, Shaner, and Eckman (1999) recently published a book containing detailed instructions on conducting substance-focused skills training sessions for people with schizophrenia and substance use disorders. The teaching approach was adapted to the learning deficits often seen in people with schizophrenia by recommending that information be repeated in different ways, that skills be practiced in various environments, and that rewards be provided for learning new skills. It utilized key concepts from Marlatt's relapse prevention approach, such as identifying high-risk situations and balancing one's lifestyle. Concepts from harm reduction and stages of change models were incorporated as well. Specific sessions were offered on identifying high-risk situations and warning signs, coping with craving, drink/drug refusal, and increasing "healthy pleasures" and social support for sobriety. The effectiveness of the approach described by Roberts, Shaner, and Eckman is under investigation, but it appears to be a promising adaptation of coping skills therapy to the treatment of persons with schizophrenia and substance use disorders.

This brief review of literature on treatment of individuals with substance abuse and schizophrenia has noted several examples of treatment manuals employing a coping skills training approach. This approach should be delivered as part of a comprehensive treatment plan that may also include case management, pharmacotherapy, money management, and motivational interviewing. The approach may have to be adapted to cognitive impairment among these individuals by emphasizing behavioral rather than cognitive coping skills, and by repetition of instruction and repeated practice of new skills.

In summary, the following is recommended for adapting cognitive-behavioral alcohol treatment for clients with comorbid alcohol dependence and psychotic disorders:

- Emphasize basic social skills building sessions (e.g., conversational skills, nonverbal behavior, developing social support networks, drink refusal skills, giving and receiving positive feedback).
- Enhance social supports and structuring of time (developing social support networks, increasing pleasant activities).
- Utilize harm-reduction and motivational interviewing approaches for clients who are not in an action stage of change.

PERSONALITY DISORDERS

Personality disorders, especially those designated as Cluster B (antisocial, borderline, histrionic, and narcissistic), are generally associated with poor response to treatment for substance use disorders (Verheul, van den Brink, & Ball, 1998). Although the specific mechanisms are largely unknown, provocative or disagreeable behaviors by these individuals may precipitate stressful life events and diminish social supports, thereby making substance use more likely. In addition, these clients tend to be noncompliant with treatment recommendations and less able than others to develop an effective working alliance with the therapist (Verheul, van den Brink, & Hartgers, 1998). Finally, these individuals may be especially vulnerable to negative affect, generally the most common relapse precipitant (Kadden, 1996), and may be poorly equipped to cope with negative emotions. However, in this regard, Woody, McLellan, Luborsky, and O'Brien (1985) found that although antisocial personality disorder alone was a predictor of poor treatment outcome, the presence of depression allowed patients to benefit from psychotherapy despite their sociopathy.

For personality-disordered clients, treatment focused solely on reducing or eliminating substance use is seldom sufficient, because their concomitant problems are likely to persist and constitute a major relapse liability. Therefore, the personality disorder needs to be addressed to contain or reduce acting-out behavior that may contribute to relapse risk. Given the long-standing nature of personality disorders and the difficulty modifying them, change efforts of this sort require continuing attention long after abstinence has been established. In the context of substance abuse treatment, a reasonable strategy is to utilize skills training to achieve some degree of behavioral change by addressing the most salient negative and disruptive features of personality functioning. In many cases, this will involve anger management training (Lewis, 1990), with a focus on the negative consequences of angry behavior, as a means of motivating a desire to change.

For clients with both alcoholism and antisocial personality disorder, Mandell (1981) recommended the use of a highly structured treatment approach, and described specific behavioral and cognitive-behavioral interventions for each of three client subtypes: primary, hysteroid, and undersocialized sociopaths. The use of a structured cognitive-behavioral approach with sociopathic clients was empirically supported in two independent patient–treatment matching studies: Both Kadden, Cooney, Getter, and Litt (1989) and Longabaugh et al. (1994) demonstrated that structured cognitive-behavioral interventions are superior for sociopathic clients compared to relationship-focused treatments. However, these findings were not replicated in Project MATCH (1997), in which cognitive-behavioral treatment was not superior to either a motivationally oriented intervention or a 12-step-oriented intervention among sociopathic clients.

Walker (1992) recommended structured cognitive-behavioral group therapy for clients with both substance dependence and a Cluster B personality disorder. He proposed that the intervention should seek to focus clients on identifying problem behaviors and their effects on themselves and others, accepting responsibility for them, and attempting to change them. He provided guidelines for the content, style, and structure of these interventions with Cluster B clients.

Linehan (1993a) described a comprehensive cognitive-behavioral program for treating borderline personality disorder, with a primary focus on decreasing suicidal behaviors and managing the crises that precipitate them. A secondary target is therapy-interfering behaviors, such as inattentiveness, lack of collaboration with the therapist, noncompliance, and various forms of limits testing. Behavioral skills training is provided in the areas of developing distress tolerance, identifying and modulating negative emotions, increasing positive events, enhancing interpersonal effectiveness, problem solving, self-management, decision making, communication skills, and relapse prevention, as well as various cognitive restructuring procedures. A therapy manual (Linehan, 1993b) provides detailed, session-by-session instructions for training these psychosocial skills in a manner not unlike our manual, including emphases on presenting new skills in small steps, providing modeling of skills, in-session rehearsal of skills, and promoting generalization of skills to clients' natural environments. The treatment is highly structured, both overall and within individual sessions. Although this treatment approach did not originally focus on alcohol or drug abuse, which are very common among clients with borderline personality disorder, more recently Linehan et al. (1999) described a modification of the program for use with clients who also have substance use disorders. Additions include substance-oriented relapse prevention training, replacement medication pharmacotherapy, and interventions to enhance the alliance between client and therapist. The program involves 1 year of weekly individual and group sessions. There are also weekly meetings among the therapists aimed at reducing staff burnout. In a clinical trial, drug-dependent borderline females randomly assigned to this approach had significantly greater reductions in substance use, greater retention in treatment, and greater improvements in social and global adjustment at follow-up than those assigned to treatment as usual. There were significant reductions in suicide attempts and anger among both groups.

In a recent development, Ball (1998) assembled a treatment manual designed specifically for those with combined substance use and personality disorders, based on findings that cognitive-behavioral therapy is a promising approach for both types of disorder. The manual combines relapse prevention techniques from the alcoholism literature and schema-focused cognitive therapy (focusing on clients' core maladaptive beliefs) adapted from the personality disorders literature. When problematic beliefs/schemas are triggered, attempts to reduce associated negative affect often involve maladaptive behaviors that impede meeting clients' basic needs. Substance use is more likely following the occurrence of these schemas and their attendant maladaptive coping attempts. Substance use may also be triggered by relapse precipitants such as those identified by Marlatt and Gordon (1985), which include negative affect, interpersonal conflict, and social pressure—precipitants to which personality-disordered clients may be especially sensitive. The proposed dual focus schema therapy is a 24-week intervention that utilizes self-monitoring, problem solving, and coping skills training to treat both the addictive and personality disorders.

Although there has been less work on treatments for dual diagnosis problems involving personality disorders than for the Axis I disorders that tend to occur with substance abuse/dependence, a few cognitive-behavioral intervention packages have been developed that hold considerable promise. A common recommendation among them is the need for structured treatment. Some of the more frequently recommended treatment elements include the following:

- Modulating negative emotions (e.g., managing negative thinking, anger management).
- Increasing positive events (increasing pleasant activities).
- Enhancing interpersonal effectiveness (e.g., assertiveness, giving constructive criticism, receiving criticism, giving and receiving positive feedback, anger management).
- Problem solving and decision making (problem solving, seemingly irrelevant decisions).
- Relapse prevention coping skills training (e.g., drink refusal skills, managing urges to drink, cue exposure with the urge-specific coping skills training).

Additional work is needed to evaluate the efficacy of this array of interventions and determine their effectiveness in clinical settings.

TOBACCO DEPENDENCE ISSUES

For clients with alcohol and substance use disorders, tobacco dependence is the most prevalent and lethal comorbid condition (Abrams, 1995; Monti, Rohsenow, Colby, & Abrams, 1995). Many persons recovering from alcohol or other drug dependence, who maintain years of abstinence from alcohol and other drugs, will die prematurely of a tobacco-related disease if they continue to use tobacco products (Hurt et al., 1996). From 71 to 97% of adults with a history of alcohol dependence are tobacco dependent, and alcoholics smoke more heavily than nonalcoholics do (Battjes, 1988; Istvan & Matarazzo, 1984; Kozlowski, Skinner, Kent, & Pope, 1989). Because tobacco use is the single most preventable cause of disability burden, chronic disease, and death, without exception, its treatment should be addressed at every opportunity, as recommended by the evidence-based Clinical Practice Guideline (U.S. Dept of Health and Human Service [USDHHS] Agency for Health Research and Quality [AHRQ]; Fiore et al., 2000).

Providing a complete clinical protocol for identifying, evaluating, motivating, and treating tobacco dependence is beyond the scope of this book. A companion book in the Guilford list provides the clinical tools for a range of treatments that can meet the needs of providers and programs with different levels of resources available—from brief motivational treatment to intensive combined cognitive-behavioral and pharmacological treatments for patients with and without psychiatric comorbidity (Abrams et al., in press). Although, ideally, the most intensive treatments are desirable for those with comorbidity, given that more alcohol/substance abusers will die or be disabled by their tobacco abuse than by their alcohol/substance abuse, any level of treatment (even obtaining only a 1 or 2% improvement in efficacy over no-treatment controls) is better than nothing at all.

Tobacco use treatment should be an integral part of any type of substance abuse program for several additional reasons. First, contrary to previously held beliefs, continued tobacco use does not help clients with alcohol or other drug disorders to stay abstinent (Sobell, Sobell, & Kozlowski, 1995). Possible reasons include bidirectional conditioning, because drinking and smoking often occur together (Shiffman & Balabanis, 1995; Abrams et al., 1992), and nicotine and alcohol operate on common brain reward pathways such as the dopaminergic system (Abrams, 1999). Second, studies demonstrated better drinking outcomes among alcoholics who quit smoking within 6 months of quitting drinking than among those who did not (Bobo, Gilchrist, Schilling, Noach, & Schinke, 1987; Sobell et al., 1995; Miller, Hedrick, & Taylor, 1983). Third, more alcohol/other drug users will die from diseases related to their tobacco use than from their alcohol/other drug use (Hurt et al., 1996). A synergistic tobacco–alcohol effect operates, conferring substantially greater risk for oral, pharyngeal, laryngeal, and esophageal cancers, and cardiovascular diseases relative to just smoking, just drinking, or neither (e.g., Centers for Disease Control, 1994a; Bosetti et al., 2000).

Timing of Tobacco Dependence/Smoking Cessation Intervention

Smoking cessation does not deleteriously affect sobriety, regardless of when it is delivered (Bobo et al., 1995; Hughes, 1995; Sobell et al., 1995). An intervention that took place early in recovery—while clients were still in residential treatment (Bobo, 1995)—provides reassurance that a voluntary, motivationally tailored intervention can be delivered and accepted by staff and patients without negatively impacting sobriety.

Interestingly, our early work (Colby et al., 1994) suggested that among alcoholic smokers, only 28% said they were contemplating cessation in the next 6 months. However, 1 month later, at the transition to outpatient care, more than 50% reported considering cessation. Early in outpatient treatment (i.e., after detoxification, inpatient, or day hospital programs) may be an opportune and "teachable" moment for treating tobacco dependence among clients with substance use disorders. Delaying treatment can result in fewer patients participating in smoking interventions (Burling, Marshall, & Seidner, 1991). In a recent pilot study with random assignment (Kalman et al., 2001), we found that fewer patients who had been assigned to a delayed versus a concurrent (with alcohol treatment) treatment actually began our smoking program (67% vs. 100%). Clearly, efforts to reduce barriers to participation may be needed to enhance engagement among patients who opt for delayed smoking treatment. It is recommended that all smokers in alcohol/substance abuse treatment be identified, motivated, and treated for tobacco dependence, either simultaneously or as soon as possible after admission.

Motivation to Quit Tobacco Use

Motivating clients with alcohol and other drug use disorders to quit cigarettes is challenging. There are patient, provider, delivery system, and cultural resistances to quitting, due in part to fear of undermining sobriety. Studies confirm that the majority of clients are not motivated to quit within 6 months of alcohol treatment (Bobo, Walker, Lando, & McIlvain, 1995; Snow, Prochaska, & Rossi, 1992). Among those in day treatment, a study in our laboratory found that 72% of clients were not planning to quit in the next 6 months (Colby et al., 1994). These rates are not very different from those of smokers in the general population, where 70% say they want to quit smoking at some point in time, but the vast majority (80%) are not ready to quit within the next 30 days (Velicer et al., 1995).

A proactive, tailored approach is recommended to reach out to smokers along the whole continuum of motivation (from least to most ready to quit). Treatment of smoking is initiated by first assessing motivation or readiness to quit. A number of tools are available to assess motivation, including the smoking contemplation ladder (Biener & Abrams, 1991) and the long and short forms of the stages of change instruments for smoking (Snow et al., 1992). Generally, someone who is not ready to make a quit attempt in the next 30 days should be given a motivational enhancement intervention (Miller & Rollnick, 2002) specifically designed for smokers (e.g., Colby et al., 1998). For a complete clinical guide to motivating smokers to quit see Emmons et al. (in press).

As in the treatment of other addictions, smokers' cognitions—especially their self-efficacy and their outcome expectancies—form the cornerstone of understanding treatment success (Abrams & Niaura, 1987; Bandura, 1997). Beyond the smoking-specific expectancies, there is a need to examine clients' beliefs and expectancies regarding how smoking and drinking influence each other. An Alcohol and Smoking Interaction Expectancies Questionnaire (Colby et al., 1994) was given to alcoholic smokers to assess their beliefs about the interaction of smoking and drinking during periods of use, and the expected effects of smoking and smoking cessation on urge to drink and recovery. Over 70% believed it would be harder to stay sober if they quit smoking. At times, 58% said they smoked to cope with an urge to drink. Reluctance to consider smoking cessation was greater among those with high levels of tobacco dependence. These results suggest reasons why some alcoholics might be resistant to smoking cessation. Such beliefs and expectations should be elicited as part of an initial assessment of patients who smoke, so that motivational enhancement counseling can be tailored to address directly clients' "myths and misperceptions" (e.g., the erroneous belief that smoking helps maintain abstinence from drinking or using hard drugs). Generally, a decision-making analysis weighing the individual pros of continuing to smoke versus the cons of smoking (or the pros of quitting and the cons of quitting) can provide a basis for modifying the attitudes, beliefs, and expectations of clients, in order to move them from considering quitting in the distant future to setting a quit date within 30 days (Emmons, in press).

Another factor that may decrease interest in cessation is greater tobacco dependence. We found that reluctance to consider smoking cessation was greater among those with higher levels of dependence. This belief may be accurate. Predictors of successful smoking cessation among stably sober alcoholics were a shorter history of smoking and less tobacco dependence (Patten, Martin, Calfas, Lento, & Wolter, 2001). This suggests that less dependent smokers may be receptive to smoking interventions and that more dependent smokers will need more intensive motivational counseling.

For alcoholics early in treatment (in their first month of sobriety), with greater levels of tobacco dependence or a stated disinterest in considering smoking cessation, a different approach may be needed. In two studies currently underway (principal investigators Abrams and Rohsenow) with recruited smokers who just entered intensive substance abuse treatment, one to three sessions of either brief advice to quit smoking using the AHRQ guideline (Fiore et al., 2000) or of motivational interviewing has resulted in 15–30% of the alcoholics' abstinence from tobacco at 1 month. Although preliminary, these results indicate that it is useful to provide at least brief advice to quit smoking, along with access to helpful pamphlets on smoking cessation, and to use nicotine replacement therapy if more intensive treatments cannot be done.

Quitting and Relapse Prevention: Cognitive-Behavioral and Pharmacological Interventions

For those who are motivated to quit smoking in the next 30 days, the best outcomes are achieved with a combination of cognitive-behavioral and pharmacological interventions (Abrams et al., in press). Evaluated self-help guides that follow a cognitive-behavioral model are available, including the American Lung Association's freedom from smoking and maintenance series. Both over-the-counter and prescription pharmacotherapies also have telephone hotlines and counseling support services that are based on cognitive-behavioral principles. The World Wide Web also now has many resources for smoking cessation. However, there is no substitute for intensive group and/or individual, face-to-face counseling of the same type and intensity used for other refractory addictions. There is a clear dose–response relationship between positive outcomes and number of treatment sessions and length of time spent within each session (DHHS-AHRQ; Fiore et al., 2000).

Cognitive-Behavioral Coping Skills

The core interventions for smoking cessation are very similar to those for alcohol and substance abuse. They include teaching cognitive-behavioral coping skills for quitting, providing skills training for coping with the acute withdrawal during the first 14 days following the quit day, and breaking the learned connections between a variety of cues and smoking. In addition, coping skills are taught for relapse prevention, as is the importance of social support during follow-up. The first 3 months after cessation is the period of highest risk for relapse, after which the risk diminishes but remains for at least the first 1–2 years and up to 5 years.

For cognitive-behavioral treatment, it is best to take a history of smoking patterns and past quit attempts, degree of nicotine dependence (Fagerstrom Tolerance Questionnaire; Fagerstrom & Schneider, 1989), personal and situational triggers for smoking (e.g., when stressed, feeling down or bored, when watching TV, driving, on the phone). Coping skills training can then be tailored to the specific high-risk situations and/or reasons why people smoke. The basic idea is to break the learned or conditioned connections between situations, intrapersonal and interpersonal, and tobacco use, and develop alternative coping skills to deal with triggers, urges, and cravings (especially during the first 2 weeks after cessation, when withdrawal symptoms are most intense). Clients are also taught other ways to achieve desired consequences without the use of tobacco products (e.g., how to alleviate stress and deal with anger, boredom, social anxiety, or depression) in healthier ways. A listing of specific active treatment components and evidence for their efficacy is outlined in detail in Abrams et al. (in press) and in the clinical practice guideline (Fiore et al., 2000).

Pharmacological Interventions

Pharmacological interventions for smokers with comorbid alcohol, other drug, psychiatric, and/or personality disorders require a professional assessment by a specialist in both mental health and addiction medicine. Pharmacological therapies may be especially important, because the chances of a current psychiatric comorbidity (e.g., depression) among tobacco users who are also alcohol/other drug abusers is extremely high. Impulse control disorders, both behavioral under- and overcontrol (e.g., adult attention-deficit/hyperactivity disorder, conduct disorder) may also be more prevalent in this population. Nicotine also alters the bioavailability of other medications, so all medications should be carefully monitored and, if necessary, adjusted (Goldstein, in press). An individual attempting to stop smoking may be discontinuing their "self-medication" for the first time since early adolescence. Neither professionals nor the client him/herself may ever have had an opportunity to be aware of the client's true "psychiatric status" without nicotine in his/her system. The underlying problems may have been masked or attenuated due to tobacco abuse. Some smokers may become severely disorganized or depressed as they cut down on cigarettes and/or try to quit for more than a few hours, and a few clients may become suicidal. Such people usually rapidly relapse back to heavy smoking or stop short of actually quitting to alleviate the emergence of these symptoms. This difficulty with past or current quit attempts and inability to delay smoking in certain circumstances may be signs of both severe nicotine dependence and as yet undiagnosed comorbidity that will need to be carefully addressed, both for the client's overall well-being and before successful cessation (or long-term sustained abstinence from alcohol or other drugs, for that matter) can be achieved.

Nicotine replacement and other pharmacotherapy products include over-the-counter and/or prescription medications such as nicotine gum or patch, inhaler, nasal spray, or the antidepressant Wellbutrin (Zyban). There are contraindications for some therapies; for example, Wellbutrin (Zyban) is known to lower the seizure threshold among alcohol abusers.

Treatment Effectiveness

Bobo et al. (1995) conducted a pilot study in residential treatment facilities involving motivational plus self-help treatment versus control. The intervention comprised 15 minutes of counseling toward the end of treatment. Of potentially eligible smoking patients, a remarkable 93% agreed to enroll in the study, and 90% completed 6-month follow-up. The intervention was well accepted by staff and patients, in part because it was tailored to the setting and was patient-centered. Bobo, McIlvain, Lando, Walker, and Leed-Kelly (1998) conducted a randomized trial in 12 residential drug treatment centers ($N = 575$). They compared a low postsmoking cessation intervention program to usual care and found that their intervention significantly improved *alcohol* abstinence at 6- and 12-month follow-up, but there were no differences on either illicit drug or tobacco use. However, participants were about twice as likely as controls to quit smoking at 6-months follow-up (8% vs. 4%) and 43% versus 40% had made a quit attempt. This study, with a large sample size and rigorous follow-up, provides strong evidence that counseling alcoholics in treatment to quit smoking may help and certainly does not jeopardize alcohol or illicit drug use outcomes. However, this low intensity tobacco dependence treatment produced very modest quit rates.

Recent studies demonstrate that more intensive, formal cessation programs produce promising results. Burling, Seidner-Burling, and Lantini (2001) compared an intensive tobacco dependence treatment alone (IT), IT with generalization training to alcohol/other substance abuse (IT + G), and usual care (UC) in 150 alcohol/drug-dependent smokers in a residential veterans treatment home. Continuous smoking abstinence at 12-month follow-up was 12% for IT, 10% for IT + G, and 0% for UC. The IT condition also had better continuous alcohol/drug use abstinence at 12 months (40%) compared to 33% in UC, and 20% in IT + G, partially replicating the Bobo et al. (1998) study that smoking cessation treatment may improve drinking/drug use outcomes when provided separately from (in parallel with) alcohol/drug treatment (IT), but *not* when the generalization of smoking cessation treatment to alcohol/other drugs is made explicit in the treatment (IT + G). Moreover, of particular interest is the result that those who were continuously abstinent from alcohol/other drugs at 12 months were continuously abstinent from smoking at the astounding rates of 29% (IT) and 50% (IT + G) versus 0% and 3%, respectively, among the subgroup of patients who were not alcohol/drug free. These rates are comparable to the best treatment outcome results reported among tobacco users who do not have alcohol/drug comorbidity (Fiore et al., 2000).

In another well-controlled study, Martin et al. (1997) recruited volunteers (sober at least 3 months) from the AA community. Participants reported a mean of 4.2 years of sobriety from alcohol. Results at 12-month follow-up revealed a cessation rate of 27%, with no differences between a standard care behavioral treatment group and two enhanced care groups (plus exercise or plus nicotine replacement). Patten et al. (1998) provide preliminary evidence that smokers with histories of both alcohol dependence and major depressive disorder can be treated with cognitive-behavioral therapy plus mood management or cognitive-behavioral therapy alone, with abstinence from smoking outcomes of 46% and 25% at 6 months, respectively, and 46% versus 12%, respectively, at 12 months. Hurt et al. (1995) provided smoking treatment to volunteers on an addictions unit and compared the results to those who volunteered for a control group. After 1 year, 12% of the treated and 0% of the untreated smokers were abstinent.

Conclusions

Early studies of tobacco dependence treatment among alcohol/substance abusers reported mixed results and have limitations in terms of methods, design, and generalizability. More recent studies are encouraging and indicate that it is possible to achieve outcomes comparable to those of studies with smokers who do not have alcohol/substance abuse comorbidity. Identifying the unique cognitive-behavioral profiles and needs of alcohol/substance abusers who are tobacco dependent may help improve treatment efficacy (Burling, Ramsey, Seidner, & Kando, 1997; Kalman, 1998). However, a range of interventions exist, from minimal (brief screening) to maximal intensity inpatient programs. A large public health benefit of reduced disease burden, death, and improved quality of life will accrue to every alcohol/substance abuser who can be encouraged to quit, whether the overall efficacy is 1% or 40% above no-treatment controls on a population basis. More intensive combined cognitive-behavioral and pharmacological treatments (Abrams et al., in press) appear better than less intensive treatments, and no treatment appears to undermine alcohol/drug use abstinence. In fact, there is increasing evidence that smoking treatment may improve alcohol abstinence rates.

Tobacco dependence treatments are both clinically and cost-effective relative to other medical and disease prevention efforts. Continued use of tobacco products is lethal and may undermine treatment of alcohol and other drug use disorders, and certainly will not help maintain a client's abstinence from alcohol or other drugs. Because tobacco dependence is more frequent among alcohol- and drug-dependent persons than any other comorbid condition and using tobacco is the single most preventable cause of disease burden, disability, and untimely death, its successful treatment should be considered a matter of necessity at any opportunity that the health care system comes in contact with clients with alcohol and other drug use disorders.

References

Abrams, D. B. (1995). Integrating basic, clinical and population research for alcohol tobacco interactions. In J. B. Fertig & J. P. Allen (Eds.), *Alcohol and tobacco: From basic science to clinical practice* (National Institute on Alcohol Abuse and Alcoholism, Research Monograph 30, pp. 281–294). Bethesda, MD: National Institutes of Health.

Abrams, D. B. (1999). Transdisciplinary concepts and measures of craving. *Addiction, 95*(Suppl. 2), S237–S246.

Abrams, D. B., Binkoff, J. A., Zwick, W. R., Liepman, M. R., Nirenberg, T. D., Munroe, S. M., & Monti, P. M. (1991). Alcohol abusers' and social drinkers' responses to alcohol-relevant and general situations. *Journal of Studies on Alcohol, 52,* 409–414.

Abrams, D. B., & Niaura, R. S. (1987). Social learning theory of alcohol use and abuse. In H. Blane & K. Leonard (Eds.), *Psychological theories of drinking and alcoholism* (pp. 131–180). New York: Guilford Press.

Abrams, D. B., Niaura, R. S., Brown, R. A., Emmons, K. M., Goldstein, M. G., & Monti, P. M. (in press). *Nicotine dependence: An evidence-based clinical guide.* New York: Guilford Press.

Abrams, D. B., Rohsenow, D. J., Niaura, R. S., Pedraza, M., Longabaugh, R., Beattie, M., Noel, N., & Monti, P. M. (1992). Smoking and treatment outcome for alcoholics: Effects on coping skills, urge to drink, and drinking rates. *Behavior Therapy, 23,* 283–297.

Abrams, D. B., & Wilson, G. T. (1986). Habit disorders: Alcohol and tobacco dependence. In A. J. Frances & R. E. Hales (Eds.), *American Psychiatric Association annual review* (Vol. 5, pp. 606–626). Washington, DC: American Psychiatric Press.

Abueg, F. R., & Fairbank, J. A. (1992). Behavioral treatments of posttraumatic stress disorder and co-occurring substance abuse. In P. A. Saigh (Ed.), *Posttraumatic stress disorder: A behavioral approach to assessment and treatment* (pp. 111–146). Boston: Allyn & Bacon.

Ahles, T. A., Schlundt, D. G., Prue, D. M., & Rychtarik, R. G. (1983). Impact of aftercare arrangements on the maintenance of treatment success in abusive drinkers. *Addictive Behaviors, 8,* 53–58.

American Psychiatric Association. (1994). *Diagnostic and statistical manual of mental disorders* (4th ed.). Washington, DC: Author.

Anthenelli, R. M., & Schuckit, M. A. (1993). Affective and anxiety disorders and alcohol and drug dependence: Diagnosis and treatment. *Journal of Addiction Disease, 12,* 73–87.

Anton, R. F., Romach, M. K., Kranzler, H. R., Pettinati, H., O'Malley, S., & Mann, K. (1996). Pharmacotherapy of alcoholism: Ten years of progress. *Alcoholism: Clinical and Experimental Research, 20* (Suppl.), pp. 172A–175A.

Azrin, N. H., Sisson, R. W., Meyers, R., & Godley, M. (1982). Alcoholism treatment by disulfiram and community reinforcement therapy. *Journal of Behavior Therapy and Experimental Psychiatry, 13,* 105–112.

Ball, S. A. (1998). Manualized treatment for substance abusers with personality disorders: Dual focus schema therapy. *Addictive Behaviors, 23,* 883–891.

Bandura, A. (1969). *Principles of behavior modification.* New York: Holt, Rinehart & Winston.

Bandura, A. (1977). *Social learning theory.* Englewood Cliffs, NJ: Prentice-Hall.

Bandura, A. (1997). *Self-efficacy: The exercise of control.* New York: Freeman.

Barlow, D. H., & Lehman, C. L. (1996). Advances in the psychosocial treatment of anxiety disorders: Implications for national health care. *Archives of General Psychiatry, 53,* 727–735.

Barnes, G. M. (1977). The development of adolescent drinking behavior: An evaluative review of the impact of the socialization process within the family. *Adolescence, 12,* 571–591.

Battjes, R. J. (1988). Smoking as an issue in alcohol and drug abuse treatment. *Addictive Behaviors, 13,* 225–230.

Beck, A. T., Rush, A. J., Shaw, B. F., & Emery, G. (1979). *Cognitive therapy of depression.* New York: Guilford Press.

Beck, A. T., Ward, C. H., Mendelson, M., Mock, J., & Erbaugh, J. (1961). An inventory for measuring depression. *Archives of General Psychiatry, 4,* 561–571.

Beck, A. T., Wright, F. D., Newman, C. F., & Liese, B. S. (1993). *Cognitive therapy of substance abuse.* New York: Guilford Press.

Bedell, J. R., Archer, R. P., & Marlowe, H. A. (1980). A description and evaluation of a problem solving skills training program. In D. Upper & S. M. Ross (Eds.), *Behavioral group therapy: An annual review.* Champaign, IL: Research Press.

Biddle, B. J., Bank, B. J., & Marlin, M. M. (1980). Social determinants of adolescent drinking: What they think, what they do and what I think they do. *Journal of Studies on Alcohol, 41,* 215–241.

Biener, L., & Abrams, D. B. (1991). The contemplation ladder: Validation of a measure of readiness to consider smoking cessation. *Health Psychology, 10,* 360–365.

Blakey, R., & Baker, R. (1980). An exposure approach to alcohol abuse. *Behaviour Research and Therapy, 18,* 319–325.

Bobo, J. K., Gilchrist, L. D., Schilling, R. F., II, Noach, B., & Schinke, S. P. (1987). Cigarette smoking cessation attempts by recovering alcoholics. *Addictive Behaviors, 12,* 209–215.

Bobo, J. K., McIlvain, H. E., Lando, H. A., Walker, D. A., & Leed-Kelly, A. (1998). Effect of smoking cessation counseling on recovery from alcoholism: Findings from a randomized community intervention trial. *Addiction, 93,* 877–887.

Bobo, J. K., Walker, R. D., Lando, H. A., & McIlvain, H. E. (1995). Enhancing alcohol control with counseling on nicotine dependence: Pilot study findings and treatment recommendations. In J. B. Fertig & J. P. Allen (Eds.), *Alcohol and tobacco: From basic science to clinical practice* (National Institute on Alcohol Abuse and Alcoholism, Research Monograph 30, pp. 225–238). Bethesda, MD: National Institutes of Health.

Bosetti, C., Franceschi, S., Levi, F., Negri, E., Talamini, R., & Vecchia, C. L. (2000). Smoking and drinking cessation and the risk of oesophageal cancer. *British Journal of Cancer, 83,* 689–691.

Brickman, P., Rabinowitz, V. C., Karuza, J., Coates, D., Cohn, E., & Kidder, L. (1982). Models of helping and coping. *American Psychologist, 37,* 368–384.

Brown, R., & Lichtenstein, E. (1979). *Relapse prevention: A non-smoking maintenance program.* Unpublished treatment manual, University of Oregon, Eugene, OR.

Brown, R. A., Evans, D. M., Miller, I. W., Burgess, E. S., & Mueller, T. I. (1997). Cognitive-behavioral treatment for depression in alcoholism. *Journal of Consulting and Clinical Psychology, 65,* 715–726.

Brown, R. A., & Lewinsohn, P. M. (1984). *Coping with depression: Course workbook.* Eugene, OR: Castalia Press.

Brown, S. A., & Schuckit, M. A. (1988). Changes in depression among abstinent alcoholics. *Journal of Studies on Alcohol, 49,* 412–417.

Burling, T. A., Marshall, G. D., & Seidner, A. L. (1991). Smoking cessation for substance abuse inpatients. *Journal of Substance Abuse, 3,* 269–276.

Burling, T. A., Ramsey, T. G., Seidner, A. L., & Kando, C. S. (1997). Issues related to smoking cessation among substance abusers. *Journal of Substance Abuse, 9,* 27–40.

Burling, T. A., Seidner-Burling, A. S., & Latini, D. (2001). A controlled smoking cessation trial for substance-dependent inpatients. *Journal of Consulting and Clinical Psychology, 69,* 295–304.

Carey, K. B. (1996). Substance use reduction in the context of outpatient psychiatric treatment: A collaborative, motivational, harm reduction approach. *Community Mental Health Journal, 32,* 291–306.

Carey, K. B., Cocco, K. M., & Correia, C. J. (1997). Reliability and validity of the Addiction Severity Index among outpatients with severe mental illness. *Psychological Assessment, 9,* 422–428.

Carey, K. B., & Correia, C. J. (1998). Severe mental illness and addiction: Assessment considerations. *Addictive Behaviors, 23,* 735–748.

Carroll, K. M. (1996). Relapse prevention as a psychosocial treatment: A review of controlled clinical trials. *Experimental and Clinical Psychopharmacology, 4,* 46–54.

Caudill, B. D., & Marlatt, G. A. (1975). Modeling influences in social drinking: An experimental analogue. *Journal of Consulting and Clinical Psychology, 43,* 405–415.

Centers for Disease Control and Prevention. (1994a). Surveillance for smoking-attributable mortality and years of potential life lost, by state—United States, 1990. *Morbidity and Mortality Weekly Report, 43,* 1–8.

Centers for Disease Control and Prevention. (1994b). Reasons for tobacco use and symptoms of nicotine withdrawal among adolescent and young adult tobacco users—United States, 1993. *Morbidity and Mortality Weekly Report, 43,* 745–750.

Chaney, E. F., O'Leary, M. R., & Marlatt, G. A. (1978). Skill training with alcoholics. *Journal of Consulting and Clinical Psychology, 46,* 1092–1104.

Childress, A. R. (1993, September). *Using active strategies to cope with cocaine cue reactivity: Preliminary treatment outcomes.* Paper presented at the NIDA Technical Review Meeting, "Treatment of Cocaine Dependence: Outcome Research," Bethesda, MD.

Childress, A. R., McLellan, A. T., Ehrman, R., & O'Brien, C. P. (1988, June). *Conditioned craving and arousal in cocaine addiction: A preliminary report.* Paper presented at the National Institute on Drug Abuse CPDD Meeting, Philadelphia, PA.

Childress, A. R., McLellan, A. T., & O'Brien, C. P. (1985). Assessment and extinction of conditioned withdrawal-like responses in an integrated treatment for opiate dependence. In L. S. Harris (Ed.), *Problems of drug dependence, 1984* (National Institute on Drug Abuse Research Monograph 55, pp. 202–210). Washington, DC: U.S. Government Printing Office.

Chung, T., Langenbucher, J., Labouvie, E., Pandina, R. J., & Moos, R. H. (2001). Changes in alcoholic patient's coping responses predict 12-month treatment outcomes. *Journal of Consulting and Clinical Psychology, 69,* 92–100.

Colby, S. M., Monti, P. M., Barnett, N. P., Rohsenow, D. J., Weissman, K., Spirito, A., Woolard, R. H., & Lewander, W. J. (1998). Brief motivational interviewing in a hospital setting for adolescent smoking: A preliminary study. *Journal of Consulting and Clinical Psychology, 66,* 574–578.

Colby, S. M., Monti, P. M., Rohsenow, D. J., Sirota, A. D., Abrams, D. B., & Niaura, R. S. (1994). *Alcoholics' beliefs about quitting smoking during alcohol treatment: Do they make a difference?* Paper presented at the annual meeting of the Research Society on Alcoholism, Maui, HI.

Collins, R., Parks, G., & Marlatt, G. (1985). Social determinants of alcohol consumption: The effects of social interaction and model status on the self-administration of alcohol. *Journal of Consulting and Clinical Psychology, 53,* 189–200.

Cooney, N. L., Bastone, E. C., Schmidt, P. M., Litt, M. D., Bauer, L. O., & Kadden, R. (1993). Cue exposure treatment for alcohol dependence: Process and outcome results. In P. Monti (Chair), *Cue exposure and alcohol treatment: Where do we stand?* Symposium conducted at the Sixth International Conference on Treatment of Addictive Behaviors, Santa Fe, NM.

Cooney, N. L., Kadden, R. M., Litt, M. D., & Getter, H. (1991). Matching alcoholics to coping skills or interactional therapies: Two-year follow-up results. *Journal of Consulting and Clinical Psychology, 59,* 598–601.

Cooney, N. L., Litt, M. D., Gaupp, L., & Schmidt, P. M. (1989, November). Recent attempts to increase alcohol cue reactivity in alcoholics: The effect of negative moods. In D. J. Rohsenow (Chair), *Recent advances in cue reactivity research in the addictions.* Symposium presented at the Annual Meeting of the Association for Advancement of Behavior Therapy, Washington, DC.

Cooney, N. L., Litt, M. D., Morse, P. A., Bauer, L. O., & Gaupp, L. (1997). Alcohol cue reactivity, negative-mood reactivity, and relapse in treated alcoholic men. *Journal of Abnormal Psychology, 106,* 243–250.

Cornelius, J. R., Salloum, I. M., Ehler, J. G., Jarrett, P. J., Cornelius, M. D., Perel, J. M., Thase, M. E., & Black, A. (1997). Fluoxetine in depressed alcoholics: A double-blind, placebo-controlled trial. *Archives of General Psychiatry, 54,* 700–705.

Dawe, S., & Powell, J. H. (1995). Cue exposure treatment in opiate and cocaine dependence. In D. C. Drummond, S. T. Tiffany, S. Glautier, & R. Remington (Eds.), *Addictive behaviour: Cue exposure theory and practice* (pp. 197–209). New York: Wiley.

Dean, L., Dubreuil, E., McCrady, B. S., Paul, C. P., & Swanson, S. (1983). *Problem Drinkers Project Manual.* Unpublished manuscript, Butler Hospital, Providence, RI.

Deas-Nesmith, D., Brady, K. T., & Myrick, H. (1998). Drug abuse and anxiety disorders. In H. R. Kranzler & B. J. Rounsaville (Eds.). *Dual diagnosis and treatment* (pp. 20–221). New York: Marcel Dekker.

Depue, J. (1982). Getting a little help from your friends. In J. Depue (Ed.), *Managing stress* (Pawtucket Heart Health Program treatment manual, pp. 1–9). Pawtucket, RI: Memorial Hospital.

DiClemente, C. C. (1991). Motivational interviewing and the stages of change. In W. R. Miller & S. Rollnick (Eds.), *Motivational interviewing: Preparing people to change addictive behavior* (pp. 191–213). New York: Guilford Press.

DiClemente, C. C., & Hughes, S. O. (1990). Stages of change profiles in outpatient alcoholism treatment. *Journal of Substance Abuse, 2,* 217–235.

Drake, R. E. (1996). Substance use reduction among patients with severe mental illness. *Community Mental Health Journal, 32,* 311–314.

Drake, R. E., Bartels, S. J., Teague, G. B., Noordsy, D. L., & Clark, R. E. (1993). Treatment of substance abuse in severely mentally ill patients. *Journal of Nervous and Mental Disease, 181,* 606–611.

Drake, R. E., Osher, F. C., Noordsy, D. L., Hurlbut, S. C., Teague, G. B., & Beaudette, M. S. (1990). Diagnosis of alcohol use disorders in schizophrenia. *Schizophrenia Bulletin, 16,* 57–67.

Drummond, D. C., & Glautier, S. (1994). A controlled trial of cue exposure treatment in alcohol dependence. *Journal of Consulting and Clinical Psychology, 62,* 809–817.

D'Zurilla, T. J., & Goldfried, M. R. (1971). Problem solving and behavior modification. *Journal of Abnormal Psychology, 78,* 107–126.

Ellis, A. (1975). *The new guide to rational living.* New York: Harper & Row.

Ellis, A., & Harper, R. A. (1961). *A guide to rational living.* Hollywood, CA: Wilshire.

Emery, G. (1981). *A new beginning: How to change your life through cognitive therapy.* New York: Simon & Schuster.

Emmons, K. M. (in press). Increasing motivation to stop smoking. In D. B. Abrams, R. S. Niaura, R. A. Brown, K. M. Emmons, M. G. Goldstein, & P. M. Monti, *Nicotine dependence: An evidence-based clinical guide.* New York: Guilford Press.

Epstein, E. E., & McCrady, B. S. (1998). Behavioral couples treatment of alcohol and drug use disorders: Current status and innovations. *Clinical Psychology Review, 18,* 689–711.

Eriksen, L., Björnstad, S., & Götestam, K. G. (1986). Social skills training in groups for alcoholics: One-year treatment outcome for groups and individuals. *Addictive Behaviors, 11,* 309–329.

Fagerstrom, K. O., & Schneider, N. (1989). Measuring nicotine dependence: A review of the Fagerstrom Tolerance Questionnaire. *Journal of Behavioral Medicine, 12,* 159–182.

Ferrell, W. L., & Galassi, J. P. (1981). Assertion training and human relations training in the treatment of chronic alcoholics. *International Journal of the Addictions, 16,* 959–968.

Finney, J. W., & Monahan, S. C. (1996). The cost-effectiveness of treatment for alcoholism: A second approximation. *Journal of Studies on Alcoholism, 29,* 229–243.

Finney, J. W., Noyes, C. A., Coutts, A. I., & Moos, R. H. (1998). Evaluating substance abuse treatment process models: I. Changes on proximal outcome variables during 12-step and cognitive-behavioral treatment. *Journal of Studies on Alcoholism, 59,* 371–380.

Fiore, M. C., Bailey, W. C., Cohen, S. J., Dorfman, S., Fox, B., & Goldstein, M. (2000). Brief clinical interventions. In *Treating tobacco use and dependence* (pp. 25–35). Washington, DC: U.S. Department of Health and Human Services.

Foa, E. B., & Kozak, M. J. (1986). Emotional processing of fear: Exposure to corrective information. *Psychological Bulletin, 99,* 20–35.

Freedberg, E. J., & Johnston, W. E. (1978). *The effects of assertion training within the context of a multi-modal alcoholism treatment program for employed alcoholics.* Toronto: Addiction Research Foundation.

Fuller, R. K., Branchey, L., Brightwell, D. R., Derman, R. M., Emrick, C. D., Iber, F. L., James, K. E., Lacoursiere, R. B., Lee, K. K., Lowenstam, I., Maany, I., Neiderhiser, D., Nocks, J. J., & Shaw, S. (1986). Disulfiram treatment of alcoholism: A Veterans Administration cooperative study. *Journal of the American Medical Association, 256,* 1449–1455.

Glasser, W. (1976). *Positive addiction.* New York: Harper & Row.

Glautier, S., & Drummond, D. C. (1994). Alcohol dependence and cue reactivity. *Journal of Studies on Alcohol, 55,* 224–229.

Goldstein, M. G. (in press). Smoking cessation: Pharmacotherapy. In D. B. Abrams, R. S. Niaura, R. A. Brown, K. M. Emmons, M. G. Goldstein, & P. M. Monti, *Nicotine dependence: An evidence-based clinical guide.* New York: Guilford Press.

Grayson, J. G., Foa, E. B., & Steketee, G. (1982). Habituation during exposure treatment: Distraction vs. attention-focusing. *Behaviour Research and Therapy, 20,* 323–328.

Greeley, J. D., Swift, W., & Heather, N. (1992). Depressed affect as a predictor of increased desire for alcohol in current drinkers of alcohol. *British Journal of Addictions, 87,* 1005–1012.

Greenberger, D., & Padesky, C. A. (1995). *Mind over mood: A cognitive therapy treatment manual for clients.* New York: Guilford Press.

Grunberg, N., & Baum, A. (1985). Biological commonalities of stress and substance abuse. In S. Shiffman & T. A. Wills (Eds.), *Coping and substance use* (pp. 25–65). New York: Academic Press.

Heather, N., Brodie, J., Wale, S., Wilkinson, G., Luce, A., Webb, E., & McCarthy, S. (2000). A randomized controlled trial of moderation-oriented cue exposure. *Journal of Studies on Alcohol, 61,* 561–570.

Hedberg, A. G., & Campbell, L. (1974). A comparison of four behavioral treatments of alcoholism. *Journal of Behavior Therapy and Experimental Psychiatry, 5,* 251–256.

Hodgson, R. J. (1989). Resisting temptation: A psychological analysis. *British Journal of Addiction, 84,* 251–257.

Hodgson, R. J., & Rankin, H. J. (1976). Modification of excessive drinking by cue exposure. *Behaviour Research and Therapy, 14,* 305–307.

Hodgson, R. J., & Rankin, H. J. (1982). Cue exposure and relapse prevention. In W. M. Hay & P. E. Nathan (Eds.), *Clinical case studies in the behavioral treatment of alcoholism* (pp. 207–226). New York: Plenum Press.

Holder, H., Longabaugh, R., Miller, W. R., & Rubonis, A. V. (1991). The cost effectiveness of treatment for alcoholism: A first approximation. *Journal of Studies on Alcohol, 52,* 517–540.

Hollon, S. D., & Beck, A. T. (1994). Cognitive and cognitive-behavioral therapies. In A. E. Bergin & S. L. Garfield (Eds.). *Handbook of psychotherapy and behavior change* (pp. 428–466). New York: Wiley.

Hughes, J. R. (1995). Clinical implications of the association between smoking and alcoholism. In J. B. Ferrtig & J. P. Allen (Eds.), *Alcohol and tobacco: From basic science to clinical practice* (National Institute on Alcohol Abuse and Alcoholism, Research Monograph 30, pp. 171–185). Bethesda, MD: National Institutes of Health.

Hurt, R. D., Dale, L. C., Offord, K. P., Croghan, I. T., Hays, J. T., & Gomez-Dahl, L. (1995). Nicotine patch therapy for smoking cessation in recovering alcoholics. *Addiction, 90,* 1541–1546.

Hurt, R. D., Offord, K. P., Croghan, I. T., Gomez-Dahl, L., Kottke, T. E., Morse, R. M., & Melton, J., III. (1996). Mortality following inpatient addictions treatment: Role of tobacco use in a community-based cohort. *Journal of the American Medical Association, 275,* 1099–1103.

Intagliata, J. C. (1979). Increasing the responsiveness of alcoholics to group therapy: An interpersonal problem-solving approach. *Group, 3,* 106–120.

Irvin, J. E., Bowers, C. A., Dunn, M. E., & Wang, M. C. (1999). Efficacy of relapse prevention: A meta-analytic review. *Journal of Consulting and Clinical Psychology, 67,* 563–570.

Istvan, J., & Matarazzo, J. D. (1984). Tobacco, alcohol and caffeine use: A review of their interrelationships. *Psychological Bulletin, 95,* 301–326.

Ito, J. R., Donovan, D. M., & Hall, J. J. (1988). Relapse prevention in alcohol aftercare: Effects on drinking outcome, change process, and aftercare attendance. *British Journal of Addictions, 83,* 171–181.

Jackson, J. K., & Connor, R. (1953). Attitudes of the parents of alcoholics, moderate drinkers, and nondrinkers toward drinking. *Quarterly Journal of Studies on Alcohol, 14,* 596–613.

Johnston, L. D., O'Malley, P. M., & Bachman, J. G. (1999). *National survey results on drug use from the Monitoring the Future Study, 1975–1998.* Rockville, MD: National Institute on Drug Abuse.

Jones, S. L., Kanfer, R., & Lanyon, R. I. (1982). Skill training with alcoholics: A clinical extension. *Addictive Behaviors, 7,* 285–290.

Jones, S. L., & Lanyon, R. I. (1981). Relationship between adaptive skills and outcome of alcoholism treatment. *Journal of Studies on Alcohol, 42,* 521–525.

Kadden, R. M. (1996). Is Marlatt's relapse taxonomy reliable or valid? *Addiction, 91*(Suppl.), S139–S145.

Kadden, R. M., Carroll, K., Donovan, D., Cooney, N., Monti, P., Abrams, D., Litt, M., & Hester, R. (Eds.) (1992). *Cognitive-behavioral coping skills therapy manual: A clinical research guide for therapists treating individuals with alcohol abuse and dependence* (Vol. 3). Rockville, MD: National Institute on Alcohol Abuse and Alcoholism.

Kadden, R. M., Cooney, N. L., Getter, H., & Litt, M. D. (1989). Matching alcoholics to coping skills or interactional therapies: Posttreatment results. *Journal of Consulting and Clinical Psychology, 57,* 698–704.

Kadden, R. M., Kranzler, H. R., & Rounsaville, B. J. (1995). Validity of the distinction between "substance-induced" and "independent" depression and anxiety disorders. *American Journal on Addictions, 4,* 107–117.

Kadden, R. M., Litt, M. D., Cooney, N. L., Kabela, E., & Getter, H. (2001). Prospective matching of alcoholic clients to cognitive-behavioral or interactional group therapy. *Journal of Studies on Alcohol, 62,* 359–369.

Kalman, D. (1998). Smoking cessation treatment for substance misuses in early recovery: A review of the literature and recommendations for practice. *Substance Use and Misuse, 33,* 2021–2047.

Kalman, D., Hayes, K., Colby, S. M., Eaton, C. A., Rohsenow, D. J., & Monti, P. M. (2001). Concurrent versus delayed smoking cessation treatment for alcoholics: A pilot study. *Journal of Substance Abuse Treatment, 20,* 233–238.

Kaminer, Y., Burleson, J., & Goldberger, R. (2001, June). *Psychotherapies for adolescents with alcohol and other substance abuse: 3- and 9-month post treatment outcomes.* Paper presented at the annual meeting of the Research Society on Alcoholism, Montreal, Quebec, Canada.

Kozlowski, L. T., Skinner, W., Kent, C., & Pope, M. A. (1989). Prospects for smoking treatment in individuals seeking treatment for alcohol and other drug problems. *Addictive Behaviors, 14,* 273–278.

Leitenberg, H. (1976). Behavioral approaches to treatment of neuroses. In H. Leitenberg (Ed.), *Handbook of behavior modification and behavior therapy* (pp. 124–167). New York: Prentice-Hall.

Lewinsohn, P. M., Antonuccio, D. O., Steinmetz, J. L., & Teri, L. (1984). *The coping with depression course: A psychoeducational intervention for unipolar depression.* Eugene, OR: Castalia.

Lewinsohn, P. M., Munoz, R. F., Youngren, M. A., & Zeiss, A. M. (1986). *Control your depression* (rev. ed.). New York: Prentice-Hall.

Lewis, C. E. (1990). Alcoholism and antisocial personality: Clinical associations and etiological implications. In H. Ollat, S. Parvez, & H. Parvez (Eds.), *Progress in alcohol research: Vol. 2. Alcohol and behavior: Basic and clinical aspects* (pp. 15–37). Utrecht: VSP.

Lied, E. R., & Marlatt, G. A. (1979). Modeling as a determinant of alcohol consumption: Effect of subject sex and prior drinking history. *Addictive Behaviors, 4,* 47–54.

Linehan, M. M. (1993a). *Cognitive-behavioral treatment of borderline personality disorder.* New York: Guilford Press.

Linehan, M. M. (1993b). *Skills training manual for treating borderline personality disorder.* New York: Guilford Press.

Linehan, M. M., Schmidt, H., Dimeff, L. A., Craft, J. C., Kanter, J., & Comtois, K. A. (1999). Dialectical behavior therapy for patients with borderline personality disorder and drug dependence. *American Journal on Addictions, 8,* 279–292.

Litman, G. K., Stapleton, J., Oppenheim, A. N., Peleg, M., & Jackson, P. (1984). The relationship between coping behaviours, their effectiveness and alcoholism relapse and survival. *British Journal of Addiction, 79,* 283–291.

Litt, M. D., Cooney, N. L., Kadden, R. M., & Gaupp, L. (1990). Reactivity to alcohol cues and induced moods in alcoholics. *Addictive Behaviors, 15*, 137–146.

Longabaugh, R., & Morgenstern, J. (1999). Cognitive-behavioral coping skills therapy for alcohol dependence: Current status and future directions. *Alcohol Research and Health, 23*, 78–87.

Longabaugh, R., Rubin, A., Malloy, P., Beattie, M., Clifford, P. R., & Noel, N. (1994). Drinking outcomes of alcohol abusers diagnosed as antisocial personality disorder. *Alcoholism: Clinical and Experimental Research, 18*, 778–785.

Maisto, S. A., Carey, K. B., & Bradizza, C. M. (1999). Social learning theory. In K. E. Leonard & H. T. Blane (Eds.), *Psychological theories of drinking and alcoholism* (2nd ed., pp. 106–163). New York: Guilford Press.

Maisto, S. A., Connors, G. J., & Zywiak, W. H. (2000). Alcohol treatment, changes in coping skills, self-efficacy, and levels of alcohol use and related problems one year following treatment initiation. *Psychology of Addictive Behaviors, 14*, 257–266.

Mandell, W. (1981). Sociopathic alcoholics: Matching treatment and patients. In E. Gottheil, A. T. McLellan, & K. A. Druley (Eds). *Matching patient needs and treatment methods in alcoholism and drug abuse* (pp. 325–369). Springfield, IL: . Thomas.

Marks, I. M. (1987). *Fears, phobias and rituals: Panic, anxiety and their disorders.* New York: Oxford University Press.

Marlatt, G. A. (1985a). Cognitive assessment and intervention procedures for relapse prevention. In G. A. Marlatt & J. R. Gordon (Eds.), *Relapse prevention: Maintenance strategies in the treatment of addictive behaviors* (pp. 201–279). New York: Guilford Press.

Marlatt, G. A. (1985b). Coping and substance abuse: Implications for research, prevention, and treatment. In S. Shiffman & T. A. Wills (Eds.), *Coping and substance use* (pp. 367–386). New York: Academic Press.

Marlatt, G. A. (1985c). Relapse prevention: Theoretical rationale and overview of the model. In G. A. Marlatt & J. R. Gordon (Eds.), *Relapse prevention: Maintenance strategies in the treatment of addictive behaviors* (pp. 3–70). New York: Guilford Press.

Marlatt, G. A., Baer, J. S., Kivlahan, D. R., Dimeff, L. A., Larimer, M. E., Quigley, L. A., Somers, J. M., & Williams, E. (1999). Screening and brief intervention for high-risk college student drinkers: Results from a two-year follow-up assessment. *Journal of Consulting and Clinical Psychology, 66*, 604–615.

Marlatt, G. A., & Gordon, J. R. (Eds.). (1985). *Relapse prevention: Maintenance strategies in the treatment of addictive behaviors.* New York: Guilford Press.

Marlatt, G. A., & Rohsenow, D. J. (1980). Cognitive process in alcohol use: Expectancy and the balanced placebo design. In N. K. Mello (Ed.), *Advances in substance abuse* (Vol. 1, pp. 159–199). Greenwich, CT: JAI Press.

Martin, J. E., Calfas, K. J., Patten, C. A., Polarek, M., Hofstetter, C. R., Noto, J., & Beach, D. (1997). Prospective evaluation of three smoking interventions in 205 recovering alcoholics: One-year results of Project SCRAP-Tobacco. *Journal of Consulting and Clinical Psychology, 65*, 190–194.

McCrady, B. S., & Miller, W. R. (Eds.). (1993). *Research on Alcoholics Anonymous: Opportunities and alternatives.* New Brunswick, NJ: Rutgers Center of Alcohol Studies.

McGrath, P. J., Nunes, E. V., Stewart, J. W., Goldman, D., Agosti, V., Ocepek-Welikson, K., & Quitkin, F. M. (1996). Imipramine treatment of alcoholics with major depression: A placebo-controlled clinical trial. *Archives of General Psychiatry, 53*, 232–240.

McGue, M. (1999). Behavioral genetic models of alcoholism and drinking. In K. E. Leonard & H. T. Blane (Eds.), *Psychological theories of drinking and alcoholism* (2nd ed., pp. 372–421). New York: Guilford Press.

McHugo, G. J., Drake, R. E., Burton, H. L., & Ackerson, T. H. (1995). A scale for assessing the stages of substance abuse treatment in persons with severe mental illness. *Journal of Nervous and Mental Disease, 183*, 762–767.

McLellan, A. T., Kushner, H., Metzger, D., Peters, R., Smith, I., Grisson, G. P., Pettinati, H., & Argeriou, M. (1992). The fifth edition of the Addiction Severity Index. *Journal of Substance Abuse Treatment, 9*, 199–213.

Meisler, A. W. (1999). Group treatment of PTSD and comorbid alcohol abuse. In B. H. Young & D. D. Blake (Eds.), *Group treatments for post-traumatic stress disorder* (pp. 117–137). Philadelphia: Brunner/Mazel.

Meyer, R. E. (1986). How to understand the relationship between psychopathology and addictive disorders: Another example of the chicken and the egg. In R. E. Meyer (Ed.), *Psychopathology and addictive disorders* (pp. 3–16). New York: Guilford Press.

Miller, E. T., Kilmer, J. R., Kim, E. L., Weingardt, K. R., & Marlatt, G. A. (2001). Alcohol skills training for college students. In P. M. Monti, S. M. Colby, & T. A. O'Leary (Eds.), *Adolescents, alcohol, and substance abuse: Reaching teens through brief interventions* (pp. 183–215). New York: Guilford Press.

Miller, W. R., Brown, J. M., Simpson, T. L., Handmaker, N. S., Bien, T. H., Luckie, L. F., Montgomery, H. A., Hester, R. K., & Tonigan, J. S. (1995). What works? A methodological analysis of the alcohol treatment outcome literature. In R. K. Hester & W. R. Miller (Eds.), *Handbook of alcoholism treatment approaches: Effective alternatives* (2nd ed., pp. 12–44). Boston: Allyn & Bacon.

Miller, W. R., Hedrick, K. E., & Taylor, C. A. (1983). Addictive behaviors and life problems before and after behavioral treatment of problem drinkers. *Addictive Behaviors, 8,* 403–412.

Miller, W. R., & Rollnick, S. (2002). *Motivational interviewing* (2nd ed.): *Preparing people for change.* New York: Guilford Press.

Miller, W. R., & Tonigan, J. S. (1996). Assessing drinkers' motivation for change: The Stages of Change Readiness and Treatment Eagerness Scale (SOCRATES). *Psychology of Addictive Behaviors, 10,* 81–89.

Miller, W. R., Westerberg, V. S., Harris, R. J., & Tonigan, J. S. (1996). What predicts relapse? Prospective testing of antecedent models. *Addiction, 91*(Suppl.), S155–S171.

Moggi, F., Ouimette, P. C., Moos, R. H., & Finney, J. W. (1999). Dual diagnosis patients in substance abuse treatment: Relationship of general coping and substance-specific coping to one-year outcomes. *Addiction, 94,* 1805–1816.

Monti, P. M., Abrams, D. B., Binkoff, J. A., Zwick, W. R., Liepman, M. R., Nirenberg, T. D., & Rohsenow, D. R. (1990). Communication skills training, communication skills training with family and cognitive behavioral mood management training for alcoholics. *Journal of Studies on Alcohol, 51,* 263–270.

Monti, P. M., Abrams, D. B., Kadden, R. M., & Cooney, N. L. (1989). *Treating alcohol dependence.* New York: Guilford Press.

Monti, P. M., Colby, S., & O'Leary, T. (Eds.). (2001). *Adolescents, alcohol, and substance abuse: Reaching teens through brief interventions.* New York: Guilford Press.

Monti, P. M., Corriveau, D. P., & Curran, J. P. (1982a). Assessment of social skill in the day hospital: Does the clinician see something other than the researcher sees? *International Journal of Partial Hospitalization, 1,* 245–250.

Monti, P. M., Corriveau, D. P., & Curran, J. P. (1982b). Social skills training for psychiatric patients: Treatment and outcome. In J. P. Curran & P. M. Monti (Eds.), *Social skills training: A practical handbook for assessment and treatment* (pp. 185–223). New York: Guilford Press.

Monti, P. M., & Kolko, D. (1985). A review and programmatic model of group social skills training for psychiatric patients. In D. Upper & S. M. Ross (Eds.), *Handbook of behavioral group therapy* (pp. 25–62). New York: Plenum Press.

Monti, P. M., & Rohsenow, D. J. (1999). Coping-skills training and cue-exposure therapy in the treatment of alcoholism. *Alcohol Health and Research World, 23,* 107–115.

Monti, P. M., Rohsenow, D. J., Colby, S. M., & Abrams, D. B. (1995). Smoking among alcoholics during and after treatment: Implications for models, treatment strategies and policy. In J. B. Fertig & J. P. Allen (Eds.), *Alcohol and tobacco: From basic science to clinical practice* (National Institute on Alcohol Abuse and Alcoholism, Research Monograph 30, pp. 187–206). Bethesda, MD: National Institutes of Health.

Monti, P. M., Rohsenow, D. J., & Hutchison, K. E. (2000). Toward bridging the gap between biological, psychobiological, and psychosocial models of alcohol craving. *Addiction, 95*(Suppl. 2), S229–S236.

Monti, P. M., Rohsenow, D. J., Hutchison, K., Swift, R. M., Mueller, T. I., Colby, S. M., Brown, R. A., Gulliver, S. B., Gordon, A., & Abrams, D. B. (1999). Naltrexone's effect on cue-elicited craving among alcoholics in treatment. *Alcoholism: Clinical and Experimental Research, 23,* 1386–1394.

Monti, P. M., Rohsenow, D. J., Michalec, E., Martin, R., & Abrams, D. B. (1997). Brief coping skills treatment of cocaine abuse: Substance use outcomes at 3 months. *Addiction, 92,* 1717–1728.

Monti, P. M., Rohsenow, D. J., Rubonis, A. V., Niaura, R. S., Sirota, A. D., Colby, S. M., & Abrams, D. B.

(1993). Alcohol cue reactivity: Effects of detoxification and extended exposure. *Journal of Studies on Alcohol, 54*, 235–249.

Monti, P. M., Rohsenow, D. J., Rubonis, A., Niaura, R. S., Sirota, A. D., Colby, S. M., Goddard, P., & Abrams, D. B. (1993). Cue exposure with coping skills treatment for male alcoholics: A preliminary investigation. *Journal of Consulting and Clinical Psychology, 61*, 1011–1019.

Monti, P. M., Rohsenow, D. J., Swift, R. M, Gulliver, S. B., Colby, S. M., Mueller, T. I., Brown, R. A., Gordon, A., Abrams, D. B., Niaura, R. S., & Asher, M. K. (2001). Naltrexone and cue exposure with coping and communication skills training for alcoholics: Treatment process and one-year outcomes. *Alcoholism: Clinical and Experimental Research, 25*, 1634–1647.

Morgenstern, J., & Longabaugh, R. (2000). Cognitive-behavioral treatment for alcohol dependence: A review of evidence for its hypothesized mechanisms of action. *Addiction, 95*, 1475–1490.

Moser, A. E., & Annis, H. M. (1996). The role of coping in relapse crisis outcome: A prospective study of treated alcoholics. *Addiction, 91*, 1101–1113.

Mueser, K. T., Fox, M., Kenison, L. B., & Geltz, B. L. (1995). *The better living skills group.* Unpublished manuscript, NH-Dartmouth Psychiatric Research Center.

Niaura, R. S., Rohsenow, D. J., Binkoff, J. A., Monti, P. M., Abrams, D. A., & Pedraza, M. (1988). The relevance of cue reactivity to understanding alcohol and smoking relapse. *Journal of Abnormal Psychology, 97*, 133–152.

O'Farrell, T. J., & Fals-Stewart, W. (2000). Behavioral couples therapy for alcoholism and drug abuse. *Journal of Substance Abuse Treatment, 18*, 51–54.

O'Leary, D. E., O'Leary, M. R., & Donovan, D. M. (1976). Social skill acquisition and psychosocial development of alcoholics: A review. *Addictive Behaviors, 1*, 111–120.

O'Malley, S. S., Croop, R. S., Wroblewski, J. M., Labriola, D. F., & Volpicelli, J. R. (1995). Naltrexone in the treatment of alcohol dependence: A combined analysis of two trials. *Psychiatric Annals, 25*, 681–688.

O'Malley, S. S., Jaffe, A. J., Chang, G., Schottenfeld, R. S., Meyer, R. E., & Rounsaville, B. (1992). Naltrexone and coping skills therapy for alcohol dependence: A controlled study. *Archives of General Psychiatry, 49*, 881–887.

Oei, T. P., & Jackson, P. R.(1982). Social skills and cognitive behavioral approaches to the treatment of problem drinking. *Journal of Studies on Alcohol, 43*, 532–547.

Oei, T. P., & Jackson, P. R. (1980). Long-term effects of group and individual social skills training with alcoholics. *Addictive Behaviors, 5*, 129–136.

Orne, M. T., & Wender, P. J. (1968). Anticipatory socialization for psychotherapy: Method and rationale. *American Journal of Psychiatry, 124*, 1202–1212.

Patten, C. A., Martin, J. E., Calfas, K. J., Lento, J., & Wolter, T. D. (2001). Behavioral treatment for smokers with a history of alcoholism: Predictors of successful outcome. *Journal of Consulting and Clinical Psychology, 69*, 796–801.

Patten, C. A., Martin, J. E., Myers, M., Calfas, K. J., & Williams, C. D. (1998). Effectiveness of cognitive-behavioral therapy for smokers with histories of alcohol dependence and depression. *Journal of Studies on Alcohol, 59*, 327–335.

Pickens, R., Bigelow, G., & Griffiths, R. (1973). An experimental approach to treating chronic alcoholism: A case study and one-year follow-up. *Behaviour Research and Therapy, 11*, 321–325.

Polich, J. M., Armor, D. J., & Braiker, H. B. (1981). *The course of alcoholism: Four years after treatment.* New York: Wiley.

Prochaska, J. O., & DiClemente, C. C. (1986). Toward a competitive model of change. In W. R. Miller & N. Heather (Eds.), *Treating addictive behaviors* (pp. 3–27). New York: Plenum Press.

Project MATCH Research Group. (1997). Matching alcoholism treatments to client heterogeneity: Project MATCH posttreatment drinking outcomes. *Journal of Studies on Alcohol, 58*, 7–29.

Project MATCH Research Group. (1998). Matching alcoholism treatments to client heterogeneity: Treatment main effects and matching effects on drinking during treatment. *Journal of Studies on Alcohol, 59*, 631–639.

Raimo, E. B., & Schuckit, M. A. (1998). Alcohol dependence and mood disorders. *Addictive Behaviors, 23*, 933–946.

Rankin, H., Hodgson, R., & Stockwell, T. (1983). Cue exposure and response prevention with alcoholics: A controlled trial. *Behaviour Research and Therapy, 21,* 435–446.

Rankin, H. J. (1982). Cue exposure and response prevention in South London. In P. Nathan & W. Hay (Eds.), *Case studies in the behavioral modification of alcoholism* (pp. 227–248). New York: Plenum Press.

Regier, D. A., Farmer, M. E., Rae, D. S., Locke, B. Z., Keith, S. J., Judd, L. L., & Goodwin, F. K. (1990). Comorbidity of mental disorders with alcohol and other drug abuse: Results from the Epidemiologic Catchment Area (ECA) Study. *Journal of the American Medical Association, 21,* 2511–2518.

Roberts, L. J., Shaner, A., & Eckman, T. A. (1999). *Overcoming addictions: Skills training for people with schizophrenia.* New York: Norton.

Rohsenow, D. J., Colby, S. M., Monti, P. M., Swift, R. M., Martin, R. A., Mueller, T. I., Gordon, A., & Eaton, C. A. (2000). Predictors of compliance with naltrexone among alcoholics. *Alcoholism: Clinical and Experimental Research, 24,* 1542–1549.

Rohsenow, D. J., & Monti, R. M. (1994). *Coping skills treatment for cocaine abusers.* Unpublished manuscript, Brown University, Providence, RI.

Rohsenow, D. J., Monti, P. M., & Abrams, D. B. (1995). Cue exposure treatment for alcohol dependence. In D. C. Drummond, S. Glautier, B. Remington, & S. Tiffany (Eds.), *Addiction: Cue exposure theory and practice* (pp. 169–196). London: Wiley.

Rohsenow, D. J., Monti, P. M., Abrams, D. B., Rubonis, A. V, Niaura, R. S., Sirota, A. D., & Colby, S. M. (1992). Cue elicited urge to drink and salivation in alcoholics: Relationship to individual differences. *Advances in Behaviour Research and Therapy, 14,* 195–210.

Rohsenow, D. J., Monti, P. M., Binkoff, J. A., Liepman, M., Nirenberg, T., & Abrams, D. B. (1991). Patient-treatment matching for alcoholics in communication skills vs. cognitive-behavioral mood management training. *Addictive Behaviors, 16,* 63–69.

Rohsenow, D. J., Monti, P. M., Hutchison, K. E., Swift, R. M., Colby, S. M., & Kaplan, G. B. (2000). Naltrexone's effects on reactivity to alcohol cues among alcoholic men. *Journal of Abnormal Psychology, 109,* 738–742.

Rohsenow, D. J., Monti, P. M., Martin, R. A., Michalec, E., & Abrams, D. B. (2000). Brief coping skills treatment for cocaine abuse: Twelve month substance use outcomes. *Journal of Consulting and Clinical Psychology, 68,* 515–520.

Rohsenow, D. J., Monti, P. M., Rubonis, A. V., Gulliver, S. B., Colby, S. M., Binkoff, J. A., & Abrams, D. B. (2001). Cue exposure with coping skills training and communication skills training for alcohol dependence: Six and twelve month outcomes. *Addiction, 96,* 1161–1174.

Rohsenow, D. J., Monti, P. M., Rubonis, A. V., Sirota, A. D., Niaura, R. S., Colby, S. M., Wunschel, S. M., & Abrams, D. B. (1994). Cue reactivity as a predictor of drinking among male alcoholics. *Journal of Consulting and Clinical Psychology, 62,* 620–626.

Rohsenow, D. J., Niaura, R. S., Childress, A. R., Abrams, D. B., & Monti, P. M. (1990). Cue reactivity in addictive behaviors: Theoretical and treatment implications. *International Journal of the Addictions, 25,* 957–993.

Rohsenow, D. J., Smith, R. E., & Johnson, S. (1985). Stress management training as a prevention program for heavy social drinkers: Cognitions, affect, drinking, and individual differences. *Addictive Behaviors, 10,* 45–54.

Rosenberg, S. D., Drake, R. E., Wolford, G. L., Mueser, K. T., Oxman, T. E., Vidaver, R. M., Carrieri, K. L., & Luckoor, R. (1998). Dartmouth Assessment of Lifestyle Instrument (DALI): A substance use disorder screen for people with severe mental illness. *American Journal of Psychiatry, 155,* 232–238.

Rosenthal, R. N., & Westreich, L. (1999). Treatment of persons with dual diagnoses of substance use disorder and other psychological problems. In B. S. McCrady & E. E. Epstein (Eds.), *Addictions: A comprehensive guidebook* (pp. 439–476). New York: Oxford University Press.

Rubonis, A. V., Colby, S. M., Monti, P. M., Rohsenow, D. J., Gulliver, S. B., & Sirota, A. D. (1994). Alcohol cue reactivity and mood induction in male and female alcoholics. *Journal of Studies on Alcohol, 55,* 487–494.

Sanchez-Craig, M., & Walker, K. (1982). Teaching coping skills to chronic alcoholics in a coedeucational halfway house: I. Assessment of programme effects. *British Journal of Addiction, 77,* 35–50.

Sartory, G., Rachman, S., & Grey, S. J. (1982). Return of fear: The role of rehearsal. *Behaviour Research and Therapy, 20,* 123–133.

Sass, H., Soyka, M., Mann, K., & Zieglgansberger, W. (1996). Relapse prevention of acamprosate: Results from a placebo-controlled study in alcohol dependence. *Archives of General Psychiatry, 53,* 673–680.

Sayette, M. A., Monti, P. M., Rohsenow, D. J., Gulliver, S. B., Colby, S. M., Sirota, A. D., Niaura, R. S., & Abrams, D. B. (1994). The effects of cue exposure on reaction time in male alcoholics. *Journal of Studies on Alcohol, 55,* 629–633.

Schuckit, M. A., Tipp, J. E., Bergman, M., Reich, W., Hesselbrock, V. M., & Smith, T. L. (1997). Comparison of induced and independent major depressive disorders in 2,945 alcoholics. *American Journal of Psychiatry, 154,* 948–957.

Shiffman, S. (1984). Coping with temptations to smoke. *Journal of Consulting and Clinical Psychology, 52,* 261–267.

Shiffman, S., & Balabanis, M. (1995). Associations between alcohol and tobacco. In J. B. Fertig & J. P. Allen (Eds.), *Alcohol and tobacco: From basic science to clinical practice* (National Institute on Alcohol Abuse and Alcoholism, Research Monograph 30, pp. 17–36). Bethesda, MD: National Institutes of Health.

Shiffman, S., & Wills, T. A. (Eds.). (1985). *Coping and substance abuse.* New York: Academic Press.

Sitharthan, T., Sitharthan, G., Hough, M. J., & Kavanaugh, D. J. (1997). Cue exposure in moderation drinking: A comparison with cognitive-behavioral therapy. *Journal of Consulting and Clinical Psychology, 65,* 878–882.

Sjoberg, L., & Samsonowitz, V. (l985). Coping strategies in alcohol abuse. *Drug and Alcohol Dependence, 15,* 283–301.

Skinner, H. A., & Allen, B. A. (1982). Alcohol dependence syndrome: Measurement and validation. *Journal of Abnormal Psychology, 47,* 189–191.

Snow, M. G., Prochaska, J. O., & Rossi, J. S. (1992). Stages of change for smoking cessation among former problem drinkers: A cross-sectional analysis. *Journal of Substance Abuse, 4,* 107–116.

Sobell, M. B., Sobell, L. C., & Kozlowski, L. T. (1995). Dual recoveries from alcohol and smoking problems. In J. B. Fertig & J. P. Allen (Eds.), *Alcohol and tobacco: From basic science to clinical practice* (National Institute on Alcohol Abuse and Alcoholism, Research Monograph 30, pp. 207–224). Bethesda, MD: National Institutes of Health.

Sontag, S. (1978). *Illness as metaphor.* New York: Farrar, Straus & Giroux.

Spielberger, C. D., Gorsuch, R. L., & Lushene, R. E. (1970). *STAI Manual for the State–Trait Anxiety Inventory.* Palo-Alto, CA: Consulting Psychologists Press.

Staiger, P. K., & White, J. M. (1991). Cue reactivity in alcohol abusers: Stimulus specificity and extinction of the responses. *Addictive Behaviors, 16,* 211–221.

Steinglass, P., Bennett, L., Wolin, S., & Reiss, D. (1987). *The alcoholic family.* New York: Basic Books.

Strickler, D. P., Dobbs, S. O., & Maxwell, W. A. (1979). The influence of setting on drinking behavior: The laboratory versus the barroom. *Addictive Behaviors, 4,* 339–344.

Tiffany, S. T. (1990). A cognitive model of drug urges and drug use behavior: Role automatic and non-automatic processes. *Psychological Review, 97,* 147–168.

Upper, D., & Ross, S. M. (Eds.). (1985). *Handbook of behavioral group therapy.* New York: Plenum Press.

Vannicelli, M. (1982). Group psychotherapy with alcoholics. *Journal of Studies on Alcohol, 43,* 17–39.

Vannicelli, M. (1992). *Removing the roadblocks: Group psychotherapy with substance abusers and family members.* New York: Guilford Press.

Velicer, W. F., Fava, J. L., Prochaska, J. O., Abrams, D. B., Emmons, K. M., & Pierce, J. P. (1995). Distribution of smokers by stage in three representative samples. *Preventive Medicine, 24,* 401–411.

Verheul, R., van den Brink, W., & Ball, S. A. (1998). Substance abuse and personality disorders. In H. R. Kranzler & B. J. Rounsaville (Eds.), *Dual diagnosis and treatment: Substance abuse and comorbid medical and psychiatric disorders* (pp. 317–363). New York: Marcel Dekker.

Verheul, R., van den Brink, W., & Hartgers, C. (1998). Personality disorders predict relapse in alcoholic patients. *Addictive Behaviors, 23,* 869–882.

Volpicelli, J. R., Alterman, A. I., Hayashida, M., & O'Brien, C. P. (1992). Naltrexone in the treatment of alcohol dependence. *Archives of General Psychiatry, 49,* 876–880.

Waldron, H. B., Brody, J. L., & Slesnick, N. (2001). Integrative behavioral and family therapy for adolescent substance abuse. In P. M. Monti, S. M. Colby, & T. A. O'Leary (Eds.), *Adolescents, alcohol, and substance abuse: Reaching teens through brief interventions* (pp. 216–243). New York: Guilford Press.

Walker, R. (1992). Substance abuse and B-cluster disorders II: Treatment recommendations. *Journal of Psychoactive Drugs, 24*, 233–241.

Wells, E. A., Catalano, R. F., Plotnick, R., Hawkins, J. D., & Brattesani, K. A. (1989). General versus drug-specific coping skills and posttreatment drug use among adults. *Psychology of Addictive Behaviors, 3*, 8–21.

Wills, T. A., & Shiffman, S. (1985). Coping and substance use: A conceptual framework. In S. Shiffman & T. A. Wills (Eds.), *Coping and substance use* (pp. 3–24). New York: Academic Press.

Wittman, M. P. (1939). Developmental characteristics and personalities of chronic alcoholics. *Journal of Abnormal Psychology, 34*, 361–377.

Woody, G. E., McLellan, A. T., Luborsky, L., & O'Brien, C. P. (1985). Sociopathy and psychotherapy outcome. *Archives of General Psychiatry, 42*, 1081–1086.

Woody, G. E., McLellan, A. T., Luborsky, L., O'Brien, C. P., Blaine, J., Fox, S., Herman, I., & Beck, A. T. (1984). Severity of psychiatric symptoms as a predictor of benefits from psychotherapy: The Veterans Administration–Penn study. *American Journal of Psychiatry, 141*, 1172–1177.

Wunschel, S. M., Rohsenow, D. J., Norcross, J. C., & Monti, P. M. (1993). Coping strategies and the maintenance of change after inpatient alcoholism treatment. *Social Work Research and Abstracts, 29*, 18–22.

Yalom, I. D. (1974). Group therapy and alcoholism. *Annals of the New York Academy of Sciences, 233*, 85–103.

Yalom, I. D., Block. S., Bond, G., Zimmerman, E., & Qualls, B. (1978). Alcoholics in interactional group therapy. *Archives of General Psychiatry, 35*, 419–425.

Ziedonis, D. M., & D'Avanzo, K. (1998). Schizophrenia and substance abuse. In H. R. Kranzler & B. J. Rounsaville (Eds.), *Dual diagnosis and treatment* (pp. 427–465). New York: Marcel Dekker.

Ziedonis, D. M., & Trudeau, K. (1997). Motivation to quit using substances among individuals with schizophrenia: Implications for a motivation-based treatment model. *Schizophrenia Bulletin, 23*, 229–238.

Index

AA (Alcoholics Anonymous), 24, 37
Abstinence, group therapy and, 35–36
Abstinence-oriented cue exposure
  with interpersonal skills training,
    15–16
  studies, 14–15
Acamprosate, 18
Acceptance, of positive feedback, 54
Accusations, about drinking/drugging,
    62
Addiction Severity Index (ASI), 164
Addictive behavior model, 3
Affect, cue reactivity and, 148–149
Aggressive interpersonal style, 48, 61,
    75, 104
Agreement, with something in
    criticism, 63
Alcohol dependence, cue reactivity
    and, 149–150
Alcohol exposure method. *See*
    Beverage exposure method
Alcoholics Anonymous (AA), 24, 37
Alcohol ingestion, as cue for heavy
    drinking, 135
Alcoholism treatment outcome studies,
    meta-analyses of, 13
Alcohol-related expectancies, 4, 6
Alcohol-Specific Role Play Test, 9
Alternative behaviors
  for refusing drinks, 65
  for urge situations, 147–148
Anger
  constructive effects of, 105
  destructive effects of, 104–105
  from false accusations, 64
  management skills training
    behavior rehearsal role plays, 107
    guidelines, 105–107, 123
    modeling, 107
    practice exercise, 108, 124–125
    rationale, 104–105, 123
    therapist Tip Sheet, 123–125
  when giving criticism, 59

Antabuse (disulfiram), 16–17
Antisocial personality disorder, 171–173
Anxiety disorders
  cue exposure treatment for, 137
  cue reactivity and, 148–149
  with substance use disorders, 104,
    168–169
Appetitive responses, conditioned, 5–6
ASI (Addiction Severity Index), 164
Assertiveness
  definition of, 49
  skills training
    behavior rehearsal role play in, 50
    guidelines for, 49–50, 75
    improvement of inpatient
      treatment, 11
    modeling in, 50
    practice exercise, 50, 76
    rationale for, 48–49, 75
    therapist Tip Sheet, 75–76
Assessments, for cue exposure
    treatment, 138–140
Attentiveness
  assertiveness and, 49
  during cue exposure, 136
  in listening, 55
Attrition, 33–34, 37
Automatic thoughts, 97
Avoidance strategy, for coping with
    urges, 146

B
Balance, 104
Beck Depression Inventory, 164
Behavior
  alternatives, for urge situations,
    147–148
  change requests
    specificity of, 59
    when being pressured to drink,
      65–66
  nonverbal. *See* Nonverbal
    communication

Behavior rehearsal role plays. *See also*
    under specific coping skills
    training sessions
  feedback for, 26
  guidelines for, 24–26
  individual considerations, 39–40
  resistance to, 24–25
  scenes, generation of, 25
Beverage cues
  client's favorite alcoholic drink as, 134
  exposure to, 140, 141–142
  responders *vs.* nonresponders, 148
Beverage exposure method
  first session, 156–157
  subsequent sessions, 159–160
  for urge-specific coping skills
    training, 140, 141–142
Bidirectional conditioning, 174
Bipolar disorder, with substance use
    disorders, 169–171
"Black-and-white" thinking, 110
Blaming the event, not yourself, 112
Body language. *See* Nonverbal
    communication
Borderline personality disorder, 172
Brainstorming, 101
Breath testing, 35
Bucket principle, 57

C
Calming down, to identify triggers, 97,
    106
Catastrophizing, 109
CBI (Coping Behavior Inventory), 8
CBT. *See* Cognitive-behavioral
    treatment
CET. *See* Cue exposure treatment
Chain of responses, stopping, 134–135
Change
  behavioral requests for, 59, 65–66
  motivation for, 28
  readiness for, self-report measures
    of, 164

responsibility for, 20–21
stages of, 16
therapeutic process model of, 16
Classical learning theory, 5, 132–133
Clients
  under influence of drugs/alcohol,
    35–36
  less-motivated, 28
  relationship with therapist, 33
  on waiting lists, management of,
    34
Closed groups, *vs.* open groups, 33
Cognitive analysis and restructuring,
  97
Cognitive-behavioral treatment. *See
  also* Coping skills training
  for anxiety disorders, 168–169
  conducting, 20
  coping behaviors and, 9
  for depression, 166–168
  drinking outcomes from, 11
  efficacy of, 12–13
  for personality disorders, 171–173
  for smoking cessation intervention,
    176–177
Cognitive factors, 7
Communication
  improvement, effects of, 67
  in intimate relationships, 67
  marital, concerning drinking
    triggers, 29–30
  skills training
    effects of, 11
    importance of, 42–43, 67
    vs. sobriety education, 15
    staff, for partial hospital treatment
      programs, 31
Compliance, 27, 36
Compromise, 49, 59, 63–64
Concurrent treatments, 31
Confidence, 7, 151
Confrontation, of dual diagnosis
  clients, 165
Constructive criticism
  characteristics of, 62
  in relationship building, 67
  skills training
    behavior rehearsal role plays in,
      60–61
    guidelines for, 58–60, 84
    practice exercise, 85
    rationale for, 57–58, 84
    therapist Tip Sheet, 84–85
Control, testing, 97
Conversation
  skills training
    behavior rehearsal role plays in,
      52
    guidelines for, 51–52, 77
    modeling in, 52
    practice exercises, 52–53, 78
    rationale for, 50–51, 77
    therapist Tip Sheet, 77–78

starting and finishing on positive
  note, 59–60
Co-occurring disorders. *See* Dual
  diagnosis
Coping Behavior Inventory (CBI), 8
Coping skills. *See also* Coping skills
  training
  cue exposure treatment and, 6
  definition of, 3
  measured, drinking outcome and, 7,
    8–9
Coping skills training
  communication skills and, 42–43
  evidence base for, 10–13
  goals of, 45
  historical roots, 2–3
  including significant others, 28–30
  individuality of, 45
  interpersonal skills, 95–96
    assertiveness, 48–50
    conversation skills, 50–53
    developing social support
      networks, 70–72
    drink refusal skills, 65–66
    giving and receiving positive
      feedback, 53–55
    giving constructive criticism, 57–
      61
    listening skills, 55–57
    nonverbal communication, 45–
      48
    resolving relationship problems,
      66–69
    structure of, 43–44
  intrapersonal skills
    anger management, 104–108
    increasing pleasant activities,
      102–104
    managing negative thinking,
      108–113
    managing urges to drink, 95–99
    planning for emergencies, 115–
      116
    problem solving, 99–102
    seemingly irrelevant decisions,
      113–115
  introduction to, 44–45
  with naltrexone, 17
  with partial hospital treatment
    programs, 31
  rationale for, 8–10
  stages of change model and, 16
  vs. control procedures, 11–12
Cotherapist teams, 22–23
Counterattacking criticism, 63
Crisis situations
  coping with, 38
  handling, 115–116
  urges during, 97
Criticism
  appropriately delivered, 61
  assertive. *See* Constructive criticism
  destructive/aggressive, 60, 62

giving, of only one issue at a time,
  69
helpful. *See* Constructive criticism;
  Positive feedback
hurtful, 60
receiving about drinking, skills
  training for
    behavior rehearsal role play in,
      64
    guidelines for, 63–64, 86
    modeling in, 64
    practice exercise, 87
    rationale for, 61–62, 86
    therapist Tip Sheet, 86–87
  separating information from
    emotion in, 62
  types of, 62–63
Cue exposure treatment
  abstinence-oriented
    description of, 14–15
    with interpersonal skills training,
      15–16
  as adjunctive therapy, 134
  administration, individual *vs.* group,
    5, 18
  assessments, 138–140
  attention focus during, 136
  conceptual overview, 132–133
  development of, 5, 6
  dosage, 137–138
  effects of, 133
  evidence base for, 14–16
  goals, 140
  length/timing of, 137–138
  methodological issues, 133–138
    safety issues, 133–134
    setting, 133–134
  moderation-oriented, 14
  with naltrexone, 18
  order of cue presentation, 136
  with partial hospital treatment
    programs, 31
  passive exposure *vs.* active coping
    during, 138
  preparation for, 156
  rationale for, 8–10, 155
  session
    beverage exposure method, 156–
      157, 159–160
    imaginal exposure to trigger,
      157–158, 160–161
    starting, 156
    termination of, 158, 161
  setting, 30
  urge-specific coping skills training.
    See Urge-specific coping skills
    training
Cues
  classical learning theory and, 5–6
  elicited reactions, drinking outcome
    and, 10
  for heavy drinking, limited alcohol
    ingestion as, 135

Cues (*continued*)
   individualized *vs.* standardized, 135
   order of presentation, 136
   reactivity to
      affect and, 148–149
      alcohol dependence and, 149–150
      responders *vs.* nonresponders, 148
      treatment session length and,
         137–138
   relevant, for exposure, 134–135
   types of, 132

D

Dartmouth Assessment of Lifestyle
      Instrument (DALI), 164
Day treatment programs, 30–31
Debating, of criticism, 63
Decatastrophizing, 112
Decision making, low-risk option, 113–
   114
Defensiveness, 63
Delay, as cognitive strategy, 146
Depression
   alcoholism and, 53
   with chemical dependence, 166–168
   cue reactivity and, 148–149
   pharmacotherapy, 166
   self-help manuals, 167
   treatment interventions, 166–167
Detoxification, 3- to 5-day, 30
Distraction, 99
Disulfiram (Antabuse), 16–17
Drink alternatives, for urge situations,
   147
Drinking behavior
   parental influences on, 4–5
   peer modeling and, 4–5
   socialization and, 51
Drinking outcome
   elicited reactions to cues and, 10
   measured coping skills and, 8–9
Drinking triggers. *See* Triggers
Drinking Triggers Interview (DTI), 138
Drink refusal skills training
   guidelines, 65–66, 88
   practice exercise, 89
   rationale, 65, 88
   therapist Tip Sheet, 88–89
DTI (Drinking Triggers Interview), 138
Dual diagnosis. *See also specific co-
      occurring disorders*
   abstinence, coping skills and, 9
   confrontation and, 165
   harm reduction philosophy for, 165
   screening for, 163–164
   treatment, 165–166

E

Emergencies, planning for
   practice exercise, 116, 131
   rationale, 115–116, 130
   skills guidelines, 116, 130
   therapist Tip Sheet, 130–131

Ending conversations, 52
Escape strategy, for coping with urges,
   146
Expectancies
   alcohol-related, 4, 6
   outcome, 6, 175
   self-efficacy, 6
Expectations
   unrealistic, 112
   for the worst situations, 109–110
Eye contact, 46, 65

F

Facial expression, 46
Family sessions, 29
Feedback
   about help you receive, 71
   for behavior rehearsal role plays, 26
   positive. *See* Positive feedback
Feelings
   anger as, 104
   negative, 111
   positive, 67–68, 111–112
   sharing, 56
   stating criticism in terms of, 58
   stating positive feedback in terms
      of, 54
Focus
   in changing negative thoughts, 112
   of criticism on drinking/drugging,
      62–63
   on single critical point, 59
Food alternatives, for urge situations,
   147
Frame of reference, changing, 101
Friendships, 50, 71, 72

G

Genetic factors, 3
Goals, unrealistic, 109
Graciousness, in appreciation of
      positive feedback, 54
Group therapy. *See also under specific
      coping skills training sessions*
   absences from, 37
   alcohol/drug use and, 35–36
   attendance, 34
   confidentiality, 35
   contract, 34–36
   for coping skills training program,
      29
   interactions in, 19–20
   outpatient closed *vs.* open groups, 33
   promptness, 35
Guided imagery procedures, negative
      affect manipulation effect on
      urge, 149

H

Habituation, 50, 133
Harm reduction philosophy, 165
Head gestures, 46–47
Head nods, 46

Helpfulness, of constructive criticism, 60
Historical events, as focus of criticism,
   62–63
Homework, 27. *See also under specific
      coping skills training sessions*
"Hopefulness" statements, 112

I

Individual treatment considerations,
   39–40
Information processing theory, 6
Inpatient setting, for cue exposure
      treatment, 133
Interpersonal relationships
   conflicts, relapses and, 61
   skills training for. *See* Coping skills
      training, interpersonal skills
Interpersonal styles, 48–49, 75
Irrational beliefs, challenging, 112

L

Learning theory
   approaches based on. *See* Coping
      skills training; Cue exposure
      treatment
   stopping chain of responses and,
      134–135
Listening
   active, 69, 71
   as conversation skill, 51
   skills training, 55–57
      behavior rehearsal role plays in,
         57
      guidelines/components of, 56, 81
      modeling in, 56–57
      practice exercise, 82–83
      rationale for, 55, 81
      therapist Tip Sheet, 81–82
Loneliness, 51, 55

M

Marital distress, 29–30
MET (motivational enhancement
      therapy), 12, 13
Meta-analyses of alcoholism treatment
      outcome studies, 13
Mind reading, 67–68
Modeling. *See also under specific coping
      skills training sessions*
   individual considerations, 39
   peer, 7
   peer and parental, 4–5
Moderation-oriented cue exposure
      studies, 14
Mood
   induction, 135
   negative, 108, 109
Motivation
   for change, 28
   for smoking cessation intervention,
      175–176
Motivational enhancement therapy
      (MET), 12, 13

N

NA (Narcotics Anonymous), 37
Naltrexone (ReVia), 17–18
Name-calling, 62
Narcotics Anonymous (NA), 37
Negative consequences
   of anger, 106
   of drinking strategy, 147
Negative thinking
   identifying, 97–98, 109–110
   management skills training
      group exercise, 113
      guidelines, 109–112, 126
      practice exercise, 113, 127
      rationale, 108–109, 126
      therapist Tip Sheet, 126–127
   telling people about, 57
Nervous movements, 46–47
Nicotine–drug interactions, 177
Nonverbal communication
   assertiveness and, 49
   in improving listening skills, 56
   skills training
      behavior rehearsal role plays, 47
      guidelines for, 46–47, 73
      modeling, 47
      practice exercise, 48, 74
      rationale for, 45–46, 73
      therapist tip sheet, 73–74
   of speaker, 56

O

Observation, 51
Open groups, *vs.* closed groups, 33
Operant conditioning, 5, 6
Opiate abusers, cue exposure
      treatment for, 137
Optimism, self-fulfilling, 112
Outcome expectancies, 6, 175
Outpatient treatment
   advantages of, 32
   attrition, 37
   closed *vs.* open groups, 33
   concurrent therapy, 37–39
      considering need for, 38
      for persistent problems, 38–39
      planning for emergencies, 38
   for cue exposure treatment, 133–
      134
   engagement in, 33–34
   group therapy, ground rules, 34–36
   length of program, 36–37
   rationale for, 31–32
   session, structure of, 32
Overconfidence, 97
Overgeneralization, 109

P

Paraphrasing, 56
Parents, influence on drinking
      behavior, 4–5
Partial hospital treatment programs,
      30–31

Passive–aggressive interpersonal style,
      49, 75
Passive delay procedure, 146
Passive interpersonal style, 48, 61, 75,
      105
Past conflicts, as focus of criticism,
      62–63
Pavlovian conditioning, 5
Peer modeling, drinking behavior and,
      4–5
Personality disorders, 171–173
Personal space, 46
Personal Toolbox, 140, 143–144, 162
Pessimism, self-fulfilling, 112
Pharmacotherapy. *See also specific drugs*
   for anxiety disorders, 169
   for depression, 166
   new, 16–18
   for smoking cessation, 177
Planning
   for emergencies. *See* Emergencies,
      planning for
   pleasant activities, 103
Pleasant activities, increasing
   practice exercise, 122
   rationale, 102–103, 121
   skills guidelines, 103–104, 121
   therapist Tip Sheet, 121–122
Point of view, changing, 101
Positive addictions, 103
Positive consequences of sobriety
      strategy, 147
Positive feedback, giving and
      receiving, skills training for
   behavioral rehearsal role plays in,
      55
   guidelines for, 54, 79
   modeling in, 54–55
   practice exercise, 55, 80
   rationale for, 53–54, 79
   therapist Tip Sheet, 79–80
Positive feelings, expression of, 67–68
Positive reinforcement, 5
Positive thinking
   categories of, 111–112
   in counteracting negative thinking,
      110, 111
Posttraumatic stress disorder (PTSD),
      169
Posture, 46
Practice exercises, 27. *See also under specific
      coping skills training sessions*
Problem drinking
   anger and, 105
   dealing with criticism and, 57
Problems
   adaptation of previous solutions,
      101
   assessment of solution effectiveness,
      101
   identifying, 101
   persistent, 38–39
   recognition of, 100

selection of solution approach, 101
solution approaches, consideration
      of, 101
Problem solving skills training
   behavior rehearsal role plays, 101–102
   guidelines for, 100–101, 119
   practice exercise, 102, 120
   rationale, 99–100, 119
   therapist Tip Sheet, 119–120
Project MATCH, 12–13, 167, 172
Psychiatric disorders
   with alcoholism. *See* Dual diagnosis
   diagnosis of, 163–164
Psychotic disorders, with substance use
      disorders, 169–171
PTSD (posttraumatic stress disorder), 169

Q

Questions
   open-ended, 51
   sincere, in clarification of criticism,
      63

R

Receptiveness, to treatment, 28
Reinforcement, 5
Relabeling distress, 112
Relapse
   cues and, 6
   examination of, 36
   inquiries about, 62
   interpersonal conflicts and, 61
   minor decisions leading to, 114
   negative consequences, thinking
      about, 98
   prevention, training for, 10–11, 13
   reduction, naltrexone and, 17
Relationship building/maintaining, 53
Relationship problems
   building up of, 67
   resolving, 66–69
      behavior rehearsal role plays, 69
      modeling, 69
      practice exercise, 91
      rationale for, 67, 90
      skills guidelines for, 67–69, 90
      therapist Tip Sheet, 90–91
Resistance, to role playing, 24–25
Responses, to your conversation, 52
Restatement, 50, 63
ReVia (naltrexone), 17–18
Review sessions, 26–27
Rights, personal, 48
Role playing. *See also under specific
      coping skills training sessions*
   individual considerations, 39–40
Role reversal, 26

S

Salivation, cue-elicited, 137
Scheduling of therapy, 29
Schizophrenia, with substance use
      disorders, 169–171

Seemingly irrelevant decisions (SIDs)
    definition of, 113
    management of
        group discussion, 114–115, 128
        group exercise, 115
        practice exercise, 115, 129
        rationale, 113–114, 128
Self-awareness, 97
Self-disclosure issue, for therapists,
        23–24, 25
Self-doubts, 97
Self-efficacy, 6, 7, 175
Self-medication, 177
Self-monitoring, 97
Self-put-downs, 110
Self-reinforcement, 112
"Self-talk," negative, 108–109
Setting
    for cue exposure treatment, 133–
        134
    for homework, 27
SIDs. *See* Seemingly irrelevant
        decisions
Significant others, recruiting into
        therapy, 29
Skin conductance, 137
Slips. *See* Relapse
SLT. *See* Social learning theory
Small talk, 51
Smoking cessation intervention, 179
    cognitive-behavioral coping skills
        for, 176–177
    effectiveness, 178
    importance of, 174
    motivation for, 175–176
    reluctance, 176
    resources, 176
    self-help guides, 176
    timing of, 174–175
Sobriety
    benefits, thinking about, 98
    education, *vs.* communication skills
        training, 15
    feeling uncomfortable about, 97
Social learning theory
    as basis for alcohol treatment, active
        participation and, 21
    coping deficit model of, 8
    cue exposure treatment and, 132–
        133
    development of, 3–4
    principles
        environmental stimuli or cues,
            5–6
        modeling, 4–5
        proximal determinants, 7
        reinforcement, 5
Social support
    appreciation for, 53
    lack of, 164–165
    to others, 72–73
    recovery and, 70
    reinforcement, 5

seeking, 71–72
sober, 99
types of, 70, 71
Social support network development
        skills training
    behavior rehearsal role plays, 72
    guidelines for, 70–72, 92
    modeling, 72
    practice exercise, 72, 93–94
    rationale for, 70, 92
    therapist Tip Sheet, 92–94
Social use, of alcohol, 65
Speaker, nonverbal behaviors of, 56
Speaking, calming down before, 58
Statements
    restatement of, 50, 63
    specific/direct, 49
State–Trait Anxiety Inventory, 164
"Stinking thinking," 108
Stress
    definition of, 3
    problem drinking and, 70
    urges during, 97
Stressors, 2
Support. *See* Social support
Suspiciousness, 64

T
Talking about ourselves, 51
Therapeutic change process model, 16
Therapist
    burnout of, 23
    cotherapist teams, 22–23
    feedback, for behavior rehearsal
        role plays, 26
    guidelines for, 23–24
    relationship with client, 33
    role reversal and, 26
    self-disclosure, 23–24
    Tip Sheets. *See under specific coping
        skills training sessions*
    training, 21–22
Thinking/thoughts
    about drinking, changing, 98
    ahead, 113
    before speaking, 49
Timing
    as listening skill, 56
    of nonverbal behavior, 47
Tobacco dependence
    prevalence, 173–174
    treatment intervention. *See* Smoking
        cessation intervention
Topics
    for conversation, 51
    for partial hospital and day
        treatment programs, 30
Training, therapist, 21–22
Treatment. *See also specific treatment
        approaches*
    goals, for partial hospital and day
        treatment programs, 30
    individual considerations, 39–40

main effects, 10–12
matching studies, 12–13
outcome studies, meta-analyses of,
        13
Triggers
    of anger, 105–106
    changing/preventing, 98
    changing response to, 107
    changing thoughts about, 106
    direct, 105
    elicitation of, 151
    in environment, 96
    escaping, 98
    hierarchies of, 137
    identification of, 96, 97
    indirect, 106
    interview on, 151–152
    for negative thinking, 110
    rank-order for frequency, 151
    relevant for exposure, 134–135,
        141
    remembering life as it was, 96
    for smoking, 177
    trauma-related, 139
12-step facilitation (TSF), 12

U
Urge-specific coping skills training
    beverage exposure, 140, 141–142
    goals of, 140
    imaginal scene exposure, 142–143
    introduction for, 140–141
    practicing urge coping skills during
        exposure, 143–145
    rationale for, 140–141
    session, overview of, 140
    urge coping strategies for, 145–
        148
    urge rating scale for, 141
Urge-Specific Strategies Questionnaire
        (USSQ), 139–140, 153–154
Urges to drink
    barriers to, 157
    definition of, 141, 151
    delaying, 99
    management skills training
        group exercise, 99
        guidelines for, 98–99, 117
        practice exercise, 99, 118
        rationale for, 96–97, 117
        therapist Tip Sheet, 117–118
    monitoring, 137
    triggers for. *See* Triggers
USSQ (Urge-Specific Strategies
        Questionnaire), 139–140, 153–
        154

V
Victim, thinking of oneself as, 113
Voice, tone of, 47, 59, 65

W
Wellbutrin (Zyban), 177